PUBLIC SUPPORT FOR PRIVATE RESIDENTIAL CARE

CASH & CARE

Editors: Sally Baldwin, Jonathan Bradshaw and Robert Walker

Cash benefits and care services together make a fundamental contribution to human welfare. After income derived from work, they are arguably the most important determinants of living standards. Indeed, many households are almost entirely dependent on benefits and services which are socially provided. Moreover, welfare benefits and services consume the lion's share of public expenditure. The operation, impact and interaction of benefits and services is thus an important focus of research in social policy.

Policy related work in this field tends to be disseminated to small specialist audiences in the form of mimeographed research reports or working papers and perhaps later published, more briefly in journal articles. In consequence public debate about vital social issues is sadly ill-informed. This series is designed to fill this gap by making the details of important empirically-based research more widely available.

Public Support for Private Residential Care

JONATHON BRADSHAW
Department of Social Policy and Social Work
University of York

IAN GIBBS
Social Policy Research Unit
University of York

Avebury

Aldershot · Brookfield USA · Hong Kong · Singapore · Sydney

© Crown Copyright, 1988

Published by
Avebury
Gower Publishing Company Limited
Gower House
Croft Road
Aldershot
Hants GU11 3HR
England

Gower Publishing Company
Old Post Road
Brookfield
Vermont 05036
USA

Library of Congress Cataloging-in-Publication Data
Bradshaw, Jonathan.
  Public support for private residential care.
  (cash & care)
  Bibliography: p.
  Includes index.
  1. Old age homes--Great Britain--Case studies
  2. Old age homes--Great Britain--Finance--Case studies.
  I. Gibbs, Ian. II. Title. III. Series
HV1454.2.G7B73   1988   362.6'1'0941   88-6185

ISBN 0 566 05661 5

Printed and bound in Great Britain by
Athanaeum Press Limited, Newcastle upon Tyne

Contents

Preface

In 1984 in the face of the rapid increase in the costs of financing people in residential homes, a Joint Central and Local Government Working Party was established. Their task was to consider ways of achieving a more coherent system of financial support for residential care. Then, as now, public finance for residential care had come either from central government through supplementary benefit, or from local government via local authority social services or social work departments. Before reaching their conclusions the Working Party recommended that pilot studies should be mounted in different parts of the country to assess the care needs of elderly people entering independent residential homes and whether the charges being made were reasonable.

This book is an account of the pilot studies that were commissioned as a result by the Department of Health and Social Security. They were undertaken by the Social Policy Research Unit at the University of York. The pilot studies began in the autumn of 1986 and were based in Lothian and parts of Devon, Sefton and Clwyd. They were undertaken quickly in order to inform the deliberations of the Joint Working Party which was due to present its own report in the summer of 1987.

Few studies in the social world, not least the present one, are free from imperfections. The constraints of time and a sample of only four local authorities were obvious limitations which are discussed more fully in the text. However, the results of pilot studies have made a contribution to the general debate about financing residents in residential care.

To have completed the work on time required the cooperation and goodwill of many people. We would like to thank in particular the social workers and registration officers in the four pilot areas who worked so closely with us. An important contribution to the research was also made by staff in local DHSS offices who were responsible for drawing the sample and providing social workers with additional information.

Although we were responsible for writing up the study for publication, our task would not have been possible without the expertise of several colleagues in the Social Policy Research Unit. Dorothy Lawton and Geoffrey Hardman undertook the whole of the data analysis; Hilary Holmes and Jenny James spent long hours coding and preparing the data; and Sally Baldwin provided invaluable advice on the policy implications of the results.

Jonathan Bradshaw and Ian Gibbs
University of York

PART I
THE ASSESSMENT OF
CARE NEEDS STUDY

1 Introduction to the assessment study

Background to the research

Since 1979 there has been a massive expansion in the number of
people living in private residential care homes for the
elderly, physically handicapped and mentally disordered.   Most
of the expansion has occurred in England and Wales where the
number of places in such homes increased by 97 per cent between
1979 and 1984.   During the same period the number of places in
voluntary homes increased by 16 per cent and in local authority
homes by five per cent.   In Scotland, private homes have not
expanded so rapidly: the increase in the number of residential
places has been limited to four per cent in both the
independent and local authority sectors.   While noting the
different experience in Scotland the overall national picture
remains one of substantial expansion.   There are no figures on
the rate of growth in residential care homes since 1984 but the
Audit Commission (1986) has estimated that the rate has
continued – perhaps doubling in each year.   Support for this
assertion is contained in the provisional results of the
Quarterly Statistical Enquiry of February 1986 which show that
90,000 people in independent residential care homes and nursing
homes were being helped by supplementary benefit compared to
42,500 in December 1984.

At present there is no legal requirement for people entering
independent homes to have their need for such care assessed.

Although a few voluntary homes carry out an assessment of care needs, in the rest of the independent sector assessment is minimal and not very well developed. In a recent study of homes in Lincolnshire the Social Services Inspectorate identified several areas for improvement in local authority assessment but noted also that the process in the private sector 'was even less rigorous and professional'. In particular, there was no stated criteria and most proprietors used intuition 'according to who they felt would be most suitable for their group' (Fryer and Mountney, 1985).

Another related trend concerns the dramatic increase in public expenditure on private residential care. The rapid expansion in the numbers of people living in private residential homes has occurred at the same time as, and some observers have argued because of, changes in the regulations governing the payment of supplementary benefits to people in residential care homes. The proportion of people receiving help with their fees through supplementary benefit payments rose from 14 per cent in 1979 to 35 per cent in 1984 and has now reached 54 per cent. Before 1986 it was not possible to separate the figures for residential care homes and nursing homes. However, for both forms of care, expenditure on the supplementary benefit element rose from £6 million in 1978 to £460 million in 1986 and the Audit Commission (1986) are suggesting that there is every prospect for further rapid growth.

The latest statistical returns, which for the first time distinguish between the two sectors indicate, that 72 per cent of total expenditure was required as a contribution towards the fees of 70,000 SB claimants in residential care homes. The remaining 28 per cent of expenditure was required for the 20,000 or so SB claimants in independent nursing homes. In 1986 the average weekly SB payment to claimants in residential care homes was £90 compared to £121 for claimants in nursing homes (DHSS 1987).

The Government has responded to these pressures in a number of ways. Up to 1983 the law provided for the payment of fees commensurate with charges for ordinary board and lodging generally in the locality. There were also discretionary powers to allow a higher amount if it would have been unreasonable to expect the person to move. These were frequently employed to meet the increased charges in homes. The Government responded in 1983 by imposing local limits for various types of homes. In order to avoid forcing people out of homes the limits were set at the highest end of the local scale and the amount payable to an individual could also be supplemented by attendance allowance and by an extension to benefit. Charges began to be levelled up to the local limits and the bill for supplementary benefit for people in independent residential care and nursing homes rose nearly fivefold between 1982 and 1984. In September 1984 the Government responded once again by freezing local limits. Then in April 1985 these were replaced by national limits that differed according to the registration category of the home. The national limits have been reviewed three times since their introduction - in November 1985, July 1986 and again in April 1987.

Meanwhile more general trends began to be recognised. The rapid growth in the number of private residential homes was accompanied by a fall in the amount of local authority sponsorship of residents in independent homes which were replaced by supplementary benefit allowances. The fall in sponsorship in England and Wales over the period 1979-1984 was about 19 per cent and about nine per cent in Scotland over a similar period. Indeed many local authorities withdrew from sponsoring new cases altogether and some, more recently, from sponsoring existing cases. In fact, faced with increasing demands for other services and pressure on their resources, local authorities have begun to reconsider their whole role in the provision of residential care. With the growth of the private sector and help with fees through supplementary benefits, demand for local authority residential accommodation fell. This presented the opportunity to diversify the use of this accommodation for day care, relief care and other purposes. In some areas, as the 1984 Registered Homes Act gave new impetus to the requirement for local authorities outside of Scotland to register and inspect private homes to ensure that they reached a reasonable standard, the local authorities have closed some of their own more inadequate stock.

The discussion of expenditure considerations and the growth in the number of people entering residential care homes should not be allowed to cloud two important issues. Increasing anxiety was expressed that people might not be receiving the most appropriate form of care for their needs, and that resources were being employed ineffectively.

The need for the research

In the context of the above developments the Department of Health and Social Security (DHSS) announced in September 1984 the establishment of a joint working party with the local authority associations, under the Chairmanship of Mr Scott

Whyte. The research reported in this book emerged directly from the recommendation for pilot studies contained in their report (DHSS 1985). A second working party, under the Chairmanship of Mrs Firth, continued the work and reported in July 1987 (DHSS 1987).

The Joint Working Parties were a development of consultations that had been going on between DHSS and the local authority associations for some time. Their primary purpose was to develop a more coherent policy for supporting residents in private and voluntary homes. The first working party's terms of reference had two more specific elements: "To consider the scope for improving....

(a) the assessment of the need of clients for residential care and

(b) ensuring that charges are related to a reasonable standard of provision and represent value for money." (para. 1.7)

The first of those concerns, the focus of Part I of the present book, arose from an anxiety that with the rapid expansion in private places, the availability of supplementary benefit and the fact that social services and general practitioners were not always involved in admission to the independent sector, people were entering residential care unnecessarily. With health treatment and supporting services they might have been cared for more appropriately, and perhaps more cheaply at home.

Much of the evidence that gave rise to this anxiety stemmed from studies in local authority homes. The former director of Warwickshire SSD interviewed by Community Care, indicated that research in his own authority had shown 'that up to 40 per cent of those going into homes did not need to, neither did they want to' (Whitehouse, 1983). The Audit Commission (1985), on the basis of their survey of expert opinion, suggested that over a third of elderly people in local authority homes had been placed there inappropriately. They concluded that the money saved by social services, some 20 per cent of all spending on the elderly, could be transferred to community care. Ovenstone and Bean (1981) reported that 12 per cent of residents in their study in Nottingham could have remained in the community had there been adequate assessment and support; and a further third should have been in the care of the health authorities. Several other studies have also identified local authority residents with undetected but treatable illnesses. (Brocklehurst, et al., 1978; Cobb, 1978; Lowther and McLeod, 1974). In essence these medical studies highlight the paradox of depriving sick elderly people of effective treatment yet allowing them to occupy a place in a local authority home unnecessarily.

Studies undertaken by the Joint Unit for Social Services Research at Sheffield University found that just under a quarter of nearly 7,000 residents were rated as very independent (Booth, et al, 1982). As a follow up study Booth and Berry (1984) attempted to discover more about these very independent residents, in particular why they were admitted and whether they could have managed in other accommodation. Broadly speaking, the residents fell into four groups: those who were rightly admitted in the first place and still could not cope outside ('then and now'); those who required residential care at the time or admission but could now cope outside ('then not now'); those not in need at admission but now unable to cope outside ('not then but now'); and, finally, those who have never been in need of residential care ('not then or now'). A minority of residents classed as 'independent' either should not have been admitted in the first place, or they should have been found accommodation more suited to their needs. However, the presence of the majority of 'independent' people in residential care could be justified on the grounds of a breakdown in their social arrangements and their need for security and companionship. The four groups identified by Booth and Berry were to play a major rôle in the analysis of our own data.

Although several studies have looked at dependency levels of residents in private and voluntary residential care homes, sometimes comparing these with levels to be found in local authority homes, few have attempted to identify the extent of unnecessary admissions to the independent sector.

The second concern, the focus of Part II of the book, arose from the escalation in supplementary benefit payments and an anxiety that the payments being made by DHSS might not represent value for money. In particular there was a concern to know if homes set their fees at or around the limits regardless of whether the facilities and services on offer justified that level of charge. There was also concern to discover whether people with particularly high care needs were able to find a place within the limits. With fuller information it was hoped that advice from local authorities would provide a better way of targetting resources.

The Joint Working Party asked themselves two questions. First, given that local authorities already apply assessment procedures for admission to their own homes, was it not also desirable and practicable for these procedures to be used "to assess the needs of people seeking support from public funds to enter or remain in residential care in the independent sector?" (para. 2.12). Second, given that local authorities have considerable experience in running their own homes and negotiating charges for sponsorship in the independent sector, were they not "in a good position to offer advice on the level of charges which it would be reasonable for supplementary benefit to meet in particular cases?" (para. 2.13)

The first working party discussed both these questions in some detail and concluded in their report that assessment for admission to local authority homes should be extended to people wishing to enter residential care in the independent sector. Moreover, that local authorities' advice should also be obtained on the reasonableness of charges in a particular home or locality. However they recommended that the arrangements should first be tested out by pilot studies. It was that recommendation which led to the establishment of the study described in this volume.

The value for money, or what became known as the reasonableness of charges, aspects of the research are considered in greater detail in Part II of this book. The rest of Part I is devoted to a closer examination and analysis of the assessment of care needs study which was intended to throw light on a number of important questions:

(1) Were there people entering private residential care homes who were not in need of such care? Was the massive increase in the numbers a result of the release of pent up demand, growth in need or younger retired people exploiting SB to enter residential care homes and hotels sooner than was necessary?

(2) What proportion of people entering were assessed already by doctors, personal social services or the homes themselves?

(3) What was involved in carrying out assessments, how long did it take and how much did it cost?

(4) How confident were social workers about the assessments they made?

(5) What practical problems, if any, might be encountered?

The participating authorities

The pilot studies took place in Lothian, and parts of Devon, Sefton and Clwyd.

The four local authorities were chosen to represent different parts of Britain and within England different types of authority - a metropolitan borough and a shire county. Although the four were located in very different geographical areas of Britain they were not selected at random or chosen to represent a cross section or typical perspective. They were selected on very different criteria, namely the existence of a substantial independent residential care sector in each area and the willingness of the four authorities to participate in the pilot studies. On these grounds they must be counted as unrepresentative of the rest of the country. However, their experience of the rapid expansion in residential care provided greater opportunities for exploring the issues than would have been otherwise available. Where an authority chose to base the study in part of the county or borough this was on the basis that a sufficient number of homes was available to produce a sample and that the practical arrangements for the assessments could be set up there.

Table 1.1 presents a selection of relevant background information on the four participating areas. There then follows a brief description of each authority.

Lothian

Apart from minor differences in nomenclature - a Social Work rather than a Social Services Department, and Part IV rather than Part III homes - the major difference between Lothian and the other areas in the study is a separate legislative structure governing the regulation of private and voluntary homes. Whereas the 1984 Registered Homes Act applies to English and Welsh authorities, all residential care in Lothian and the rest of Scotland is governed by the 1968 Social Work (Scotland) Act.

The project was based in the whole of Lothian, a region covering 677 square miles and containing a population of nearly three-quarters of a million people, two thirds of whom live in Edinburgh. Social work is based in five divisions, three in Edinburgh, one in West Lothian and one covering East and Mid Lothian. The SWD employs roughly 4,800 equivalent full-time staff and has an annual budget of nearly £60 million.

Table 1.1

Background information on the four pilot areas

	Lothian	Devon	Sefton	Clwyd
1. Area in square miles	677	2591	58	937
2. Population (000's)	745	978	299	396
3. % population aged 65-74	8.3	10.7	8.9	9.7
4. % population aged 75 and over	6.3	8.7	6.9	7.2
5. Gross expenditure on elderly as % of total gross expenditure by SSD/SWD	32.6	38.7	38.9	39.5
6. Number of LA homes	26	55	18	22
7. Number of places/beds in LA homes	1258	2274	705	932
8. Number of elderly in LA homes	1150	2017	643	888
9. Number of elderly in LA homes as % of population over 75	2.5	2.4	3.1	3.1
10. Occupancy of LA homes as %	93	89	93	93
11. Gross charge per resident in LA homes (£ per week)	169	93	97	105
12. Average net expenditure per place/bed in LA homes (£ per week)	130	47	61	73
13. Average net expenditure for every person aged over 75 (£ per week)	7.91	3.89	5.55	5.16

Table constructed from following sources:
  Personal Social Services Statistics 1984-85 Actuals
  Revenue Account, Lothian Regional Council, for year to 31
      March 1986
  Statistical Unit, Scottish Office Library
  Statistical Bulletin, Social Work Services Group, Scottish
      Education Department, July 1986
  Population Estimates, Scotland, Mid-year Estimates, 30 June
      1985, Registrar General, Scotland, HMSO 1986

The region is served by seven local DHSS offices, five of which had elderly claimants who met the criteria for possible participation in the assessment study.

At the time of the study there were 32 voluntary and 18 private residential care homes in the region providing about 1,200 places. In addition, the authority has 26 of its own Part IV homes providing 1,258 places. The predominance of the voluntary sector, and the authority's long experience of sponsoring elderly people in that sector, created a very different set of circumstances from those in the other pilot areas. Lothian continues to sponsor existing residents in both the voluntary and private sectors, but has stopped sponsoring new entrants. Even so, well established procedures exist for setting and updating charges and the majority of homes have had a rate set for them by the local authority. Homes are not obliged to charge this rate - it is set as the minimum necessary for the home to provide a reasonable quality of service.

Devon

There are more elderly people in independent residential care homes in Devon than in any other part of Britain. When the overall total is adjusted for the number of residents per 1,000 population only East Sussex displaces Devon from the top of the list. Over the last ten years the number of private and voluntary homes registered with the county council has grown by 150 per cent. The 500 or so homes are registered at the present to provide 7,700 places. There are 55 Local Authority homes with 2,274 places in this region which covers 2,591 square miles and has a population of just under one million people.

At the time of the study the SSD worked within a three-tier structure composed of areas, divisions and teams - this complex structure is now in the melting pot following an extensive review of the Department by a senior management team. The impending changes are likely to place greater stress on de-centralisation with 'teams' having a greatly enhanced rôle.

Devon's four main areas, (North, South, East and West) contained, in all, eight divisions. The East Area contained in turn three of the eight divisions (East, Exeter and Tiverton). It was decided to base the study in the East Division of the East Area, a division with 77 private and six voluntary residential care homes for the elderly with over 1,400 places. The vast majority of residential care homes are found in the towns of the coastal strip that runs from Exmouth to Lyme

Regis. Exmouth, with nearly 40 homes, is by far the most popular location followed by Sidmouth with 14 homes. Although the town of Lyme Regis is in Dorset three homes in the district of Uplyme fall within the compass of East Devon Social Services.

Sefton

The Metropolitan Borough of Sefton, a creation of the 1974 re-organisation of local government, is the most northern of the five Merseyside district authorities. It covers some 58 square miles, and has a population of just over a quarter of a million. It is an unusual amalgam of traditional industrial areas such as Bootle, prosperous domitory suburbs and, further along the A565, the seaside resort of Southport.

At the time of the re-organisation of local government Sefton had 40 registered private and voluntary residential care homes. Thirteen years later that figure is now over 130, most located in the town of Southport. Crosby has also experienced a rapid increase in the number of homes opening. Sefton has more elderly residents in the independent sector than any other Metropolitan District in England. When adjustments are made for population size only four local authorities in Britain (Devon, West and East Sussex and I.O.W.) have more elderly residents than Sefton in the independent sector. There are 18 Part III homes in the area which provide 705 places.

Given the heavy concentration of homes in Southport it was decided to limit the study in Sefton to that area. Southport, one of six social services areas, is served by one local DHSS office. The town and the surrounding areas have long been popular with retired people from Merseyside, Greater Manchester and Lancashire. Many homes also advertise nationally. As a consequence many residents are admitted from outside the area covered by the SSD, a factor involving important implications for the assessment of care needs study. From an early stage in the expansion of private residential care Sefton's policy has been to foster co-operation with owners, the health service, and other council departments. They have also actively encouraged home owners to form their own local associations. The keywords in their policy are consultation, co-operation and facilitation (see Murray, 1986; Watson, 1986). While many authorities would also feel that these now reflect their own philosophy Sefton anticipated and responded to the issues at a much earlier stage.

Clwyd

The county of Clwyd, the coalescence of the former counties of Flintshire and Denbighshire, takes its name from the vale of that name and the river that meets the sea at the holiday resort at Rhyl. The county covers an area of 937 square miles and contains a population of 400,000 people. The County Council and Administrative Centre are based in the market town of Mold in the east of the county. The six social services areas, coterminous with the six district borough councils within Clwyd, employ more than 1,800 people in the various locations. The combined revenue and capital budget for the SSD is £20 million.

The study was based in the Borough of Rhuddlan whose population of 52,000 is largely concentrated on the two coastal towns of Rhyl and Prestatyn. The area is served by one social services office and one local DHSS office, around the corner from one another in the centre of Rhyl. Given its position and facilities Rhyl is a popular retirement area for elderly people from within the county and an increasing number of people from the West Midlands, Manchester and Merseyside.

There are 34 private and two voluntary homes in the borough providing 730 beds. Rhyl with 19 homes and Prestatyn with 10 are the two most favoured locations. A survey of private sector residents in 1983 had found that 80 per cent were admitted from the local area, 12 per cent from other parts of Clwyd and eight per cent from outside the county. Among the 80 per cent of 'locals' is a significant number of English people who retired to the area and then subsequently entered residential care there rather than returning to the area where they had previously lived. The county of Clwyd has 22 Part III homes with 932 places. However, the borough of Rhuddlan has a shortage of Part III accommodation and, with the imminent closure of a home for women only, long waiting lists exist for the 100 or so beds in the one remaining local authority home.

Similar to the other two areas outside of Scotland, Clwyd had no experience in assessing the reasonableness of charges in the independent sector. For their own Part III homes they calculated a unit cost based on running costs and debt charges.

For simplicity, an overall label is used when referring to the three areas where the study was based in only part of the county or borough. Thus, the East Division of the East Area of Devon, Sefton-Southport and Clwyd-Rhuddlan have been shortened to Devon, Sefton and Clwyd respectively.

Selecting and contacting the sample of elderly people

Every registered independent home for the elderly in the four areas received a letter in July 1986 from DHSS, Carey Street, London with information about the study. It was made clear that residents in that home who met certain criteria might be included in the study. The 'dry-run' nature of the study was also stressed and home owners and managers were assured that residents' entitlement to benefit would not be affected by the exercise. Table 1.2 indicates the number of homes for the elderly in the four areas and the number visited as part of the assessment of care needs study.

Table 1.2
Independent homes for the elderly in four pilot areas

Area	All homes			Homes visited for assessments		
	Private N	Voluntary N	Total N	Private N	Voluntary N	Total N
Lothian	18	32	50	11	26	37
Devon	77	6	83	67	3	70
Sefton	77	12	89	44	4	48
Clwyd	34	2	36	25	2	27
Totals	206	52	258	147	35	182

It was decided to restrict the assessments of care needs to elderly people who were by far the largest of the client groups found in residential care homes. Assessments for other groups would have introduced too many practical and research complications for such a short project. However, which elderly people to include in the sample was also the focus of considerable discussion. An ideal design for this study would have been for

(1) Potential claimants to be assessed before they entered homes, and

(2) Residents already in homes to be assessed when they claimed SB.

These may be the circumstances when assessments will be required in practice. However at the present time those who claim supplementary benefit for residential care are almost invariably already in residential homes – they cannot claim until they are. Furthermore, even if it was possible to identify potential claimants seeking to enter residential care there was not enough time to collect a sample of sufficient size. We estimated that in the three months available for fieldwork we would have obtained a sample of less than 120 entrants.

Another possibility was to select the sample for assessment from those already in residential care homes and who had been there and on SB for less than a year. However this sample alone would have limited the usefulness of the study as a means of testing the feasibility of assessing the care needs of people before they enter homes because:

(1) The health and general condition of residents may have improved, or more likely deteriorated, since being admitted.

(2) An important aspect of any assessment is to see how the person manages at home, what family and neighbourly support is available and what services might be required. Persons already in residential care may well have given up their houses and community links.

(3) Assessing people sometime after admission requires the answer to two questions. Were they in need of residential care when first admitted? Were they in need of that care when assessed at a later stage? Providing answers to the former retrospectively would have proved very difficult.

For these reasons we felt it prudent to complement assessments of those SB claimants already in care ('retrospective') with assessments of those admitted during the fieldwork period ('live'). The sample of those already in care was obtained from local supplementary benefit offices. Before final instructions for drawing the sample were issued, DHSS offices in Exeter, Southport and Rhyl were visited by a member of the research team in order to identify with staff any potential problems. For the seven offices serving the Lothian Region a joint meeting was held at the DHSS Central Office (Argyll House) in Edinburgh.

With resources available for up to 1,000 assessments in what was to be a quantitative exercise it seemed reasonable to go for the largest number in each area that could be afforded. On this basis, 250 assessments in each of the four areas could have been undertaken. However, in order to have completed the research by April 1987, in time for it to be considered by the Joint Working Party before publishing their report, we needed to limit our fieldwork to three months. For such a brief and intensive task it was necessary for the participating authorities to appoint temporary staff. Even so, during a period of three months there was a limit to the number of assessments each person could achieve, a point the authorities had stressed at an early stage. Rather than 250, a figure that looked increasingly unrealistic, each authority was asked to aim for 150 assessments during the three months. All agreed to attempt this number, although Sefton and Clwyd remained uncertain whether it was feasible in the time.

On the basis of information collected by the authorities about the number of elderly people entering private and voluntary homes in the previous years, it seemed possible that the sample would be composed of four-fifths of those already resident before 1 September 1986 and one-fifth who would enter during the fieldwork period of September, October and November.

For the 'retrospective' assessments we would have preferred the elderly person to have been in residential care for less than one year, and to have been claiming SB for residential care for a first time within this period. A 'retrospective' sample drawn on these criteria would have eased the assessor's task. However, after discussion with local DHSS offices, it was clear that applying such strict criteria would have again yielded too small a sample. The following instructions for drawing the sample, issued to local DHSS offices, were intended to overcome these difficulties:

(1)   Identify claimants over pensionable age in voluntary or private <u>residential care homes</u> (not nursing homes) who have been claiming at their current address for (a) less than 12 months in August and (b) between 12 and 24 months. Keep the two groups separate.

(2)   List all the cases identified under 1(a) on the enclosed control sheet. If this is less than 170 cases select the balance at random from group 1(b). Enter the claimant's name, CP No., and address. Where the information is readily available record the length of time the claimant has been in the home.

(3)   Select 170 cases from the list and send one of the enclosed letters to the Claimant or, if appropriate, the appointee. Enter the date of issue on the control sheet. Hold the case for two weeks.

(4) If a reply is received note on the control sheet whether the claimant/appointee has granted/refused co-operation.

(5) Two weeks after the letter has been issued to the claimant /appointee:

   (i) Send a list of claimants/appointees who have agreed to take part and those who have not replied to [name of local SSD/SWD].
   (ii) Send a copy of the control sheet to SB3D, London, with a copy of the summary.

(6) Where local resources permit, it would be appreciated if in addition to the above you could include in the study people who make enquiries at the LO about entering voluntary or private residential care. For the period 1.9.86 to 28.11.86 enquirers who are definitely known to be entering or placing a relative in voluntary or private residential care, should be issued with a letter requesting their participation. Details should be sent to the Social Services/Social Work Departments as in (4) and (5) above and copied to SB3D.

(7) Exceptionally, researchers may contact local offices direct for information on individual cases. They will provide a signed release from the claimant concerned.

Item 6 of the instructions above is a reference of course to the 'live' cases we wished to include in the sample. The earlier letter from DHSS to owners and managers had also sought their co-operation in alerting the assessors to any elderly person entering their homes during the period of fieldwork who would be claiming supplementary benefit for residential care. As a third measure, social work teams and hospital social workers were asked to pass on the names of any cases they knew of.

The achieved sample in each area

The intended sample was set at 150 assessments for each authority although, as noted above, Sefton and Clwyd felt this might not be possible in their own areas. In order to allow for some elderly people who would not wish to participate, up to 170 letters from DHSS were sent out in each area to claimants meeting the criteria for inclusion in the study. Table 1.3 sets out the number of refusals in each area.

Table 1.3

Number of claimants written to and refusals by area

RETROSPECTIVE CASES

	Written to by DHSS	Refusals		Cases sent to SSD/SWD	Cases assessed	LIVE CASES	Total of all cases
	N	N	%	N	N	N	N
Lothian	170	31	18	139	128	24	152
Devon	110	14	13	96	144	12	156
Sefton	170	39	23	131	96	16	112
Clwyd	139	28	20	111	96	14	110
Totals	589	112	19	477	464	66	530

Notes: Retrospective cases= claimants resident in home before 1.9.86
Live cases= claimants entering home after 1.9.86

In deciding the number of claimants to be contacted we had allowed for a refusal rate of about 12 per cent. In the event the rate was nearer 20 per cent, much higher than anticipated. Apart from knowing claimants' names and which home they were in we had little further useful information about those people who did not wish to participate in the study. It is difficult therefore to compare them with the rest of the sample in order to discuss possible bias. In the absence of relevant information it is not possible to know, for example, whether fitter claimants might be disproportionately more reluctant to co-operate or, conversely, whether non-participation might be higher among those incapable of handling the enquiry.

On the basis of information provided by the four authorities at the start of the study it had also been predicted that the overall sample would include about 20 per cent 'live' assessments, that is elderly people entering residential homes during the fieldwork period. Contrary to expectation this did not happen. One explanation, suggested by the assessors and confirmed by staff at local DHSS offices, was that the number of people entering homes was down on previous years. The fine autumn weather and relatively mild winter during the period of fieldwork were also mentioned as major factors.

As a consequence the final sample was composed of 87.5 per cent 'retrospective' and 12.5 per cent 'live' assessments. The experience of each area in contacting and interviewing their sample is as follows:

Lothian

The five local DHSS offices involved were able to identify 170 people who met the criteria for selection. During the two week 'waiting period' 31 people indicated their wish not to be interviewed, leaving 139 names which were forwarded to the assessors in due course. For one reason and another, including the death of one resident, 11 of the 139 names were not contacted. The remaining 128 names formed the bulk of the 'retrospective' interviews, complemented by 24 'live' assessments of people admitted to homes during the period of fieldwork. As Table 1.3 indicates a total of 152 assessments were achieved in Lothian.

Devon

It was only possible for DHSS Exeter to issue 110 letters to people who, on the basis of their records, met the criteria for inclusion in the study. Of these 14 refused straight away and a further six refused when contacted by the assessor for an appointment. Nonetheless, as Table 1.3 indicates, 156 assessments were completed in Devon. Some of the deficit was made up by 12 'live' assessments, but in the main the 'missing' names were traced by the assessor. Her long experience of working with elderly people, and contacts in residential homes in the area, enabled her to identify a further 54 claimants whose names had not been 'lifted' during the DHSS trawl. Forty of this latter group fell well within the criteria for inclusion in the study; six were just outside, that is, they had been claiming SB for up to six months beyond the cut off point of two years; and the remaining eight, in so far as they had been claiming SB for three years or longer, were well outside the criteria for inclusion. The inclusion of the 14 cases who fell outside the criteria for selection introduces a slight but, in our opinion, not too serious bias into the analysis. In order to have maintained the 'purity' of the sample they should have been excluded but the advantages of retaining them outweighed the disadvantages.

Sefton

DHSS in Southport identified and contacted 170 people meeting the criteria for inclusion but nearly one quarter refused. Although en-bloc refusal from residents in a home was a problem experienced in each area it was especially acute in Sefton. Twenty-eight of the 39 refusals were concentrated in seven homes where most, if not all, those selected declined to be interviewed. It is difficult to avoid the conclusion that some home owners and managers were actively advising their residents against participation.

Of the 131 'retrospective' names provided to Sefton Social Services Department by the local DHSS office, not all were found to be available or eligible for assessment when the home was contacted by the assessors. This was for a variety of reasons - eg. death, transfer to hospital, movement elsewhere, last-minute change of mind about participation, etc. In one case, the resident had ceased to be a supplementary benefit claimant, having sold her house.

Regarding the 'live' cases, more than 16 names were initially provided by DHSS but several had to be eliminated. For instance, in some cases it was found that the resident was only at the home on a short-term basis.

So, in Sefton a total of 112 assessments were completed, three-quarters of the number set. However, both Sefton and Clwyd, as indicated above, had stressed that given the thoroughness and complexity of their existing assessment procedures it would have been unrealistic with the resources and time available to achieve 150 interviews, even if that many names had been forwarded to them.

Clwyd

Only with one home was there any suggestion that an owner had been advising against participation, the rest of the refusals were spread fairly evenly throughout the homes contacted. Nonetheless, the number of refusals, 20 per cent of those sent the letter, was again more than had been expected. In total the assessors completed 96 'retrospective' interviews and 14 with 'live' cases. Again, for reasons similar to those outlined above for Sefton, Clwyd was only able to complete three-quarters of the target number of assessments set.

The sample: marital status, age and sex

Two-thirds of those assessed were widowed and a further 20 per cent were single (Table 1.4). Of those who were married 40 per cent were in the same residential care home as their partner, a third of partners were still living in the marital home and the others were living locally, overseas and one was in another residential care home.

Table 1.4
Marital status

Marital status	N	%
Single	107	20.2
Married	35	6.6
Widowed	356	67.2
Divorced/Separated	32	6.0
Totals	530	100.0

Married – partner in	N
Same residential home	14
Still in marital home	11
Living locally	3
Living overseas	1
Living in a different residential home	1
Total	30

Missing cases= 5

The age distribution is given in Table 1.5 There were seven men and one woman under retirement age in the sample but as would be expected the sample was in general very old – 70 per cent were over 80 including many who were over 90.

Table 1.5
Age

Age	N	%
Less than 60	4	0.8
60–64	8	1.5
65–69	27	5.1
70–74	39	7.4
75–79	87	16.4
80–84	139	26.2
85–89	134	25.3
90–99	91	17.2
100	1	0.2
Totals	530	100.0

There is a question about whether the seven men and one woman under pension age should have been included in the sample. They were all in residential homes for the elderly and all but one was receiving supplementary benefit at the limits for those in residential care homes registered for the elderly. All but one was assessed by the social workers as in need of residential care when first admitted and still in need of care ('Then and now').

Pen portraits of the cases are given below and we can find no reason to exclude them from the sample on the basis of their age.

Case 2/67 - 'Then and now'

- Male, age 57, single.
- Entered the present home in August 1986 after living alone in his own home.
- He is a diabetic - has angina - receives Invalidity Benefit and Mobility Allowance. He has a personality problem and has days of depression and wanders at night.
- Judged as not fit to live alone and advised by GP and social worker to move into residential care although he is still maintaining his flat.

Case 2/112 - 'Then and now'

- Male, age 59, widowed.
- Entered home in June 1986 after living at home with his wife who died suddenly.
- He has Motor Neurone disease and is deteriorating rapidly and will soon need full nursing/hospital care.
- His wife previously cared for him and he admitted himself into the home when she died.

Case 4/66 - 'Not then but now'

- Male, age 55, single
- Categorised as "disabled under pension age" - suffers from epilepsy and has been cared for by his parents all his life.
- Was admitted to the home with his father after living in very poor housing conditions - could have coped outside residential care if rehoused with his father and given support services.
- His father's health has now deteriorated (the son's condition has stayed the same), so when the father dies, the son's case will be reconsidered.

Case 4/128 – 'Then and now'

- Female, age 49, separated.
- Multiple sclerosis victim, chairbound, condition deteriorating.
- Chose Home 305 against medical advice and offers of places in two nursing homes. Needs total care and apparently receives it.

Case 1/13 – 'Then and now'

- Male, age 64, widower.
- Transfer from psycho-geriatric unit upon daughter's instigation.
- Alcoholic who has failed to maintain himself adequately since death of wife 2 years ago. Suffers memory loss – has tendency to wander. Mental state such that "could no longer live in the community" – his initial disturbed behaviour now controlled by MELLERYL.

Case 1/27 – 'Then and now'

- Male, age 64, separated.
- Prior to admission lived with 'frail' mother who could not cope with him – prior to that lodging houses following marriage break up.
- His mental condition (unspecified) is such that he requires constant supervision – has little or no memory – tendency to alcohol abuse.

Case 1/89 – 'Then and now'

- Male, age 63, divorced.
- Suffered stroke in Australia – returned to England to live with mentally retarded brother who couldn't provide necessary support – speech unintelligible causes severe distress – frequently depressed/suicidal.
- This home is staffed by Nuns with a liberal admission policy.

Case 2/76 – 'Then and now'

- Male, age 64, married.
- Spouse in same home.
- Stroke victim with poor sight – wife unable to cope with large house and care for husband who became aggressive following illness. Both moved into the Home where their daughter is one of the professional staff and assessed their need for care.

Table 1.6 indicates that over three-quarters of the sample were women. Nearly half the women, but only a quarter of the men, were in the 85 and over age group. Conversely, nearly a third of men, but only 10 per cent of women, were under 75 years of age.

Table 1.6
Percentage of men and women in four broad age groups

Age

Sex	64 & under		65-74		75-84		85 & over		Totals	
	N	%	N	%	N	%	N	%	N	%
Men	8	6.8	28	23.7	51	43.2	31	26.3	118	22.3
Women	4	1.0	38	9.2	175	42.5	195	47.3	412	77.7
Totals	12	2.3	66	12.5	226	42.6	226	42.6	530	100.0

$X^2 = 38.72$ $P < 0.0001$

Note: The X^2 test quoted in this and other tables must be seen as indicative because the sample is not statistically representative.

The sample: admission from where

In all, 39 per cent of the sample were first admitted to their present residential care home from hospitals - 26 per cent following a short-term or acute episode and 13 per cent after a stay in hospital of at least one month.

Table 1.7 summarises where they were living before they were first admitted to the present residential care home or hospital. Over 60 per cent were admitted from their own home including 17 per cent who were living in sheltered housing. A further 17 per cent came from the homes of relatives and 15 per cent from other residential care or nursing homes. Those who were not admitted directly from hospital were more likely to come from the homes of relatives and other private or voluntary residential care homes and less likely to be from their own home.

Of those who entered residential homes from their own home including sheltered housing, 80 per cent were living alone at the time of admission, 13 per cent were living with a spouse and six per cent with other relatives.

Table 1.7
Usual place of residence before admission

Usual place of residence	Admitted from hospital N= 209 (39%)	Not admitted from hospital N= 321 (61%)	All N= 530
Their own home (excluding sheltered housing)	51.4	40.9	45.1
Sheltered housing	19.2	14.7	16.5
The home of relatives	12.0	20.3	17.0
The home of friends/ neighbours	1.4	0.6	0.9
Another private/voluntary residential home	5.8	16.6	12.3
Local authority Part III or Part IV home	1.9	1.6	1.7
Nursing or convalescent home	0.5	1.6	1.1
Hotel, boarding house, lodgings or hostel	3.8	3.1	3.4
Long term hospital	3.8	—	1.5
Homeless	—	0.3	0.2
Religious order	—	0.3	0.2
Totals	100.0	100.0	100.0

2 Assessment and assessors

Existing arrangements for assessment

Each of the four areas in the study employ a set of procedures for assessing the care needs of elderly people. The assessment provides the basis for deciding whether to admit the person to a local authority residential home. An outline of assessment in the four areas is presented below:

Lothian

In practice this is not strictly an assessment 'for residential care' but an attempt to determine whether there exists a need for residential care or whether domiciliary and other forms of support would enable the elderly person to remain at home. The normal procedure involves the referral to a generic social worker who visits the elderly person and completes a social history and assessment, drawing, where necessary, on information from relatives, neighbours, home helps, community nurses, etc. The form used is largely 'open-ended' and invites the social worker to comment and provide details of important events and items such as previous occupation, skills, hobbies, personality traits, family relationships and attitudes. This is followed by background details covering community and domiciliary support, housing, social contacts and any reasons why the person cannot remain in the community.

The social worker then sends the form along with a covering letter to the patient's GP asking for basic information on the elderly person and giving consent to her or him being seen by a geriatrician. The social work assessment and GP's report are then sent to a consultant geriatrician who usually, though not invariably, examines the elderly person to decide whether residential care is the most appropriate course of action. The papers are then returned to the social worker who makes a recommendation which, in turn, is considered by the area team. They will then send the requests to a Divisional Panel which, having scrutinised all the relevant papers, makes a recommendation for or against the elderly person being offered a residential place. There are four divisional panels: one for Edinburgh, covering three social work divisions, one for each of the other three 'county' divisions of West, East and Mid-Lothian. In Edinburgh the panel meets centrally; in the county divisions it meets in the homes which have vacancies. Panels are chaired by an assistant principal from the social work department. Normally they will include the social worker who has made the request, representatives from the area team, a geriatrician, someone from the homes which have vacancies and someone from administration.

Quite a few voluntary homes in Lothian are known to require a medical assessment before the person is admitted. In addition, a minority of private homes offer care plans based on medical assessments.

Devon

Assessment in Devon varies considerably in the different areas of the county. At the time of the study the formal assessment was not an elaborate procedure although the North Devon Area were piloting a standard process. In the rest of the county the main documentation consists of a form (SS 112) which is, as titled, an "Application for Admission to Residential Care" rather than an assessment schedule as such. Page 1 of the form contains a number of questions covering basic background information about the elderly person, including a signed agreement by the applicant not to dispose of any resources before or after admission. The second page covers various aspects of the applicant's general health. Sufficient space is also provided for the social worker to include a brief background history with details of any particular problems, and other significant events.

In brief, Devon has a short formal application form rather than an extensive assessment schedule. However, the information collected and contained within the formal application was only part of an assessment involving a variety of informal procedures. While accepting that assessment in Devon tends to be less elaborate and is carried out more quickly than in other parts of the country, their social workers were anxious to stress that the information contained in the application form was only a partial reflection of the assessment they would have undertaken.

In principle it is possible for Form SS 112 to be complemented by information from Form SS 113 or Form SS 114 which are medical reports supplied by the elderly person's general practitioner for a set fee. In practice medical reports have not been extensively sought although this situation is likely to change in the light of Devon's own study and development of a standard process.

Assessment panels in Devon include heads of homes, home care organiser, community physician, team leader (housing), occupational therapist and social workers.

Sefton

Assessment of need for Part III accommodation involves various procedures, depending on the source of the referral, and the stage at which residential care becomes a possibility. For example, a new referral to the area team of an old person in need of services or care would involve a home visit by a social worker and assessment of the old person's needs and social circumstances, reported on a general four page form (SS1) with the title 'Casepaper'. The first two pages cover a range of basic information about the client including items on their present state of health, significant medical events and an extensive list of services required or already provided. The final two pages are set aside for a descriptive social history of the client with an instruction to the social worker to 'follow topic headings set out on the social history contents form'. Although an assessment might include opinions sought from a GP or health visitor there remains no formal medical input. Considerably more medical information would be included in an assessment from a hospital social worker, who would also use the same casepaper form, because this would be known and more readily available. The whole process of investigation and assessment of need for services and care, of necessity, takes a long time, especially when relatives have to be contacted. Area team social workers estimated that, in most cases, assessment required at least a day's concentrated work.

In addition to the general casepaper SS1, a different type of assessment procedure is in operation at a specialist assessment

/rehabilitation unit known as Chase Heys. As a residential home, Chase Heys has three main functions - assessment, short-stay care and long-stay care. The objective of the assessment made during an elderly person's short residence here, is to assess what services and facilities are required for rehabilitation to the community. Although rehabilitation to the community is an important aim, the result of the assessment period may be that long-stay residential care is required, following which the person will be admitted to another Part III establishment (or occasionally, to the Chase Heys long-stay wing should a bed be available). Emergency admissions are sometimes made to this unit.

The case papers and assessments records that are emerging from this process are more extensive, and have a formal medical input. In particular, an alternative assessment form has been developed from the work at Chase Heys. The form contains 40 questions covering background details; home circumstances prior to admission; a medical enquiry form; functional dependency ratings; services received or needed prior to admission; financial circumstances; and a final section of three questions on main sources of referral, who assessed the need for care and a social history of the elderly person. In brief, the document represents a comprehensive assessment and includes considerable overlap and coverage of the items and issues under investigation in the present research.

At the time of the research Sefton were considering how the assessment casepapers being developed at Chase Heys could be incorporated into the SS1 procedure in a way that would enhance the effectiveness of the area social worker's assessment and recording. Given that some, if not a great deal, of the Chase Heys' work was likely to become part of the normal procedures in due course it was decided to employ a modified version of the assessment form as the main Sefton instrument.

One feature of the 'actual Chase Heys' pilot assessment form (as distinct from the modified version which was used for the research study) was that it incorporated space for recording ongoing information about the person's ability to perform various self-care tasks and other aspects of dependency (mobility, continence, etc.), for each week during the initial six-week assessment period. Clearly it would not have been appropriate to have used this part of the form as it stood, in the research study. On the other hand, there were some specific questions to which answers were required for the purposes of the research study, which were not included as such on the real Chase Heys form. These included SB history and other financial details, and the questions on who assessed the need for care. In order to provide the information needed for the research, these questions were taken from the questionnaire and appended to the modified Chase Heys form. The rationale for this was that the whole assessment could be done from one form (the transfer of data to the questionnaire being completed later in the office, as instructed), while still obtaining the additional non-assessment details required for the research.

Clwyd

Until quite recently social workers in Clwyd completed a brief two page form of background information about the person who had been assessed. Similar to Devon, and perhaps the experience of other areas, the formal document was little more than a summary of some of the salient points that emerged during the assessment. The form could not be taken as a reflection of all that had taken place.

In an attempt to present assessment information in a more extensive and systematic way, and introduce a greater degree of standardisation into the assessment process, Clwyd replaced their short form with a 15 page schedule entitled 'Personal Case Sheet/Application for Residential/Day Care'. The form, the largest in use in the four areas, is a trial one. Similar to Sefton, the form was developed at a specialist assessment unit and then adapted for trials with area social work teams. Apart from being the longest it was also the most comprehensive of the forms associated with assessment. The first two pages are essentially the old form, with items covering a range of background information. Additional items seek information about family support, personal history, contacts and a detailed day by day account of services needed or received. The form includes sections, each with several, sometimes as many as a dozen, questions on self-care; mobility; vision; hearing; incontinence; behavioural problems; psychiatric and/or psychological problems; and mental confusion. The last two pages are a summary sheet for the assessment, including an Action Plan, and a review sheet with treatment goals and action.

Similar to the other areas, there was little systematic preparation or training for using the form or, indeed, for undertaking the assessment in the first place. A meeting was held in Rhyl for the area social workers to discuss the new form; the ability to carry out assessments is acquired through experience, a point endorsed by existing social workers in all areas.

The area team in Rhyl is composed of 11 generic social workers each taking one or two elderly people as part of their case load. The new form, while daunting at first sight, was found by social workers to be very thorough and helpful but requiring more than one visit to complete properly. However, given that it was standard procedure to visit the client more than once this was not a problem. Assessment approached on this basis tends to require a lot of time, in most cases at least the equivalent of a day's work, sometimes two.

Restraints, limitations and problems

Chapter 1 of this book has already discussed the characteristics of the four areas and emphasized that their experience of residential care and other factors make them untypical areas. Likewise, from a later section in this chapter, it is clear that the assessors were more qualified and experienced than would be normal in many authorities.

It should also be borne in mind that the study, covering only the elderly, was undertaken by specially appointed staff who were aware that it was a dry run exercise. The relatively brief period of fieldwork also prevented us from including as many 'live' cases in the sample as we would have liked.

The need to keep as close as possible to existing procedures was stressed many times and was given special emphasis at the briefing session held for the social work assessors. However, a certain amount of departure from the normal course proved inevitable. In Clwyd, for example, it was not unusual for Part III assessments to take as long as the equivalent of two days. Within the timescale of this study it was not possible to allow assessors that amount of time - had we done so, less than 50 assessments would have been completed. Sefton, likewise, would have managed only 70 assessments. Concessions were also necessary in Lothian who would normally carry out multi-disciplinary assessment for possible Part IV admissions, with both time and cost implications. After discussions with the social work department, multi-disciplinary assessment, with GP and geriatrician input, was limited to the 'live' admissions.

To have rigidly adhered to existing procedures in each area would have required a very different study operating over a longer period of time and with far more resources. Given the urgency that this study was required, and the funding available, practical adjustments had to be made. As a result assessments for the study of necessity differed from the form of assessment that would have been undertaken had the elderly people in the sample sought admission to local authority homes. In short, the assessments were carried out by temporary staff, without prolonged discussion with other workers, unconstrained by scarcity and without access to an alternative package of care. In spite of these restraints we believe the approach to assessment, including documentation, retained the essential features of assessment in each area.

The major organisational constraint was caused by the delay in issuing instructions to local DHSS offices for drawing the sample. In the three authorities outside of Scotland assessors did not receive the list of residents until mid-September; in Lothian the delay was more serious and assessors were unable to make a start until the beginning of October. This meant extending the original fieldwork period by two weeks, essential if the number of assessments, already below the 600 anticipated, was to be maximised.

The assessment questionnaire

Much of the research questionnaire was completed by the assessors on the basis of information they had obtained during the assessment. In addition, the assessors also provided important details about the amount of time required, those involved and other aspects concerning the process of assessment. The questionnaire was not intended to replace existing documentation in use in the four areas. In order for the assessment to remain as close to the normal pattern as possible it was essential that the relevant admittance forms or case papers were completed. The briefing for assessors had provided clear instructions to complete existing documentation first and then transfer relevant data to our questionnaire and respond to the sections that asked about the nature of assessment, how it was undertaken and what problems had been encountered. From this brief explanation it is clear that the questionnaire was not the assessment form as such but a vehicle for collecting previously recorded data and an opportunity for the assessor to reflect on the task.

The questionnaire was discussed with various interested parties at several stages in its development. Initial drafts were considered within the Social Policy Research Unit and by existing social workers and link people in the four areas. Later versions were also sent to DHSS for suggestions and comment. Last minute fine tuning was based on the comments offered by the assessors at their briefing in York. The limited amount of time available for the study prevented any opportunity for piloting the questionnaire.

The assessors

Each authority in the study made their own decision as to who should carry out the assessments. In practice three options were open to them. They could have appointed temporary staff whose sole purpose would have been to carry out the assessments for the duration of the project. A second was to spread the workload among existing social work staff. A third option was for some of the assessments to have been undertaken by existing staff and some by temporary staff. The second option was ruled out almost straight away as being both unrealistic and unreasonable. The third, whilst requiring considerably less of existing social workers, would still have increased an already demanding caseload with rushed and perfunctory assessment as a result. The first option, though not without weaknesses, was the one preferred by each authority. As a result temporary staff were appointed to work either full-time or part-time on the assessment of care needs study.

Table 2.1 indicates the number of assessors in each area and the nature of their appointment, full or part-time. Additional columns in the table provide a breakdown of the number of retrospective and live assessments completed.

Table 2.1
The assessors and number of assessments completed

Area	Assessor	Appoint-ment	Retro-spective N	Live N	Total assessments N
Lothian	1	PT	32	7	39
Lothian	2	PT	29	6	35
Lothian	3	FT	67	11	78
Devon	1	FT	144	12	156
Sefton	1	PT	53	7	60
Sefton	2	PT	43	9	52
Clwyd	1	PT	48	6	54
Clwyd	2	PT	48	8	56
Totals			464	66	530

All the assessors were women who came to the project with a wealth of social work experience. Six of the eight were graduates who also held professional social work qualifications, two were employed as unqualified social workers. One of the unqualified social workers held a nursery nurse qualification and the Institute of Welfare Officers Certificate, the other had started a social work course at a polytechnic but had withdrawn when her husband was transferred by his firm to another part of the country. All, at one time or another, had worked with the elderly either in hospitals or the community, some of the assessors had experience in both settings. They had all worked for their respective authorities on previous occasions, either in a full or part-time capacity.

From this brief outline of the assessors it is clear that we had extremely able, experienced and well qualified people working with us. They may be untypical in the sense of being too well qualified and experienced. While assessment may be carried out by unqualified and inexperienced staff in other areas of the country this was not the case, as far as we could determine, in the four pilot areas in the study. In any event we had little trouble in accepting that well qualified and experienced assessors would be a positive feature of the assessment study.

The assessors were briefed for their task in York at the beginning of September 1986. The focus of the meeting was the latest version of the research questionnaire which would be completed by the assessors after each assessment of an elderly person. Special emphasis was placed on the need for them to follow existing procedures as closely as was practically possible, including the completion of relevant documentation. It was essential that any influence of the research questionnaire on the way the assessment was carried out was kept to a minimum. Discussion during the meeting also allowed us to identify some important last minute amendments to the questionnaire. These were incorporated into a final version which assessors received 10 days later. They also received a 12 page booklet offering advice and guidance for completing the questionnaire.

Reflections from the assessors

According to the assessors, assessment for the study differed in a number of major ways from their experience of undertaking assessment in the past.

The major departure from normal practice was the lack of opportunity to visit the elderly person in their own home. This was true for all the retrospective and the vast majority of the live cases who were seen of necessity in the setting of the residential home. Assessors stressed the importance of seeing clients in their own home and, if possible, more than once. In brief, they were telling us that certain important judgements can only be made in the light of first hand impressions.

Most importantly, they would not have worked with a single client group in such a concentrated way. Elderly clients and assessment would have formed only part of a generic social workers' caseload, and even hospital based social workers in specialist geriatric units would not be expected to spend all their time on assessment. The assessors developed considerable expertise in the practice of assessment during the three months of fieldwork, and from their comments found the task enjoyable and rewarding. Although assessors acknowledged that boredom and loss of motivation might result from continual involvement in assessment they were also aware of the merits of such specialisation. In particular, a specialist worker with knowledge of services and residential care would have a better overall view. They also raised the possibility of specialist workers being given greater responsibility for registration and assessment in the independent sector. Another suggestion was for generic teams to include more specialist social workers who would be responsible for assessment, placement and support of the elderly in the community. Taken together their comments support a specialist rôle for social workers in this area.

Although the problems of keeping to normal procedures was dealt with in greater detail in an earlier section it is worth noting the assessors' views on this subject. All, including Devon, were agreed that the assessments for the study were usually less time consuming than those that would be required for admitting elderly people to local authority homes. Once assessment for the study had been completed contact with the elderly person was lost. In a live situation, as opposed to a dry-run, social workers would maintain regular contact before admission. In Lothian and some other areas, the contact would be maintained during the admission and on to the first review three months later. Assessors missed this continuity of contact with the client.

Assessors confirmed that it was easier to make assessments where the events and judgements were reasonably recent, with the proviso that the elderly person had been allowed sufficient time to adjust to the situation. Assessment too soon after painful events ran the risk of further upsetting the elderly person.

Because the majority of assessments were carried out on people already in residential care reliable information and records were not always available. Assessors in Lothian, where medical information was required for the assessment, frequently experienced difficulties in locating this information. Often when the person had been in the home for some time their medical records had been transferred by the former GP to the doctor looking after residents in the home. On other occasions the situation was further complicated when the original GP had retired or could not recall where the records had gone. Assessors in Lothian also commented that the information on the medical certificate was not necessarily the most useful, and that talking to the GP could often be more relevant.

3 The outcome of the assessment

Need for residential care

The social worker assessors were asked to allocate the elderly person to one of four categories on the basis of their assessment. The results are presented in Table 3.1. In the assessors' opinion 91.3 per cent of the whole sample needed to be in their residential homes. A further 2.1 per cent were assessed as in need of residential care when first admitted but were now able to cope outside with appropriate accommodation and support services. Therefore a total of 93.4 per cent of the overall sample were in need of residential care when first admitted. Those considered not in need of residential care at admission were divided into 2.8 per cent who were unable to cope outside any longer and 3.8 per cent who could still cope outside with appropriate accommodation and support services. However, the need for residential care was closely linked to where the person had been living or staying before their admission to their present residential care home. For example, whereas only one person (less than one per cent) admitted from hospital was judged <u>not</u> to be in need of care at the time of admission, over 11 per cent of those admitted from the community fell within this category.

Table 3.1
Need for residential care by source of admission

Source of admission

Need for care:	From hospital		From other residential care		From the community		All admissions	
	N	%	N	%	N	%	N	%
1. Then and now	203	97.1	57	90.5	224	86.8	484	91.3
2. Then not now	5	2.4	1	1.6	5	1.9	11	2.1
3. Not then but now	1	0.5	3	4.8	11	4.3	15	2.8
4. Not then or now	–	–	2	3.2	18	7.0	20	3.8
Totals	209		63		258		530	100.0

X^2= 23.30   P<0.001

Description of 4 groups:

1. **'Then and now'**: Those requiring residential care at the time of admission and still requiring care

2. **'Then not now'**: Those requiring residential care at the time of admission but now able to cope outside with appropriate accommodation and support services

3. **'Not then but now'**: Those not in need of residential care at the time of admission but now unable to cope outside even with appropriate accommodation and support services

4. **'Not then or now'**: Those not in need of residential care at the time of admission and still able to cope outside with appropriate accommodation and support services

It is important to remember that the judgement about need for residential care has to take into account not only the needs of the individual but also the availability of resources that might enable the person to continue to manage at home. Assessors made their judgements in the context of the availability of appropriate accommodation and support services in their area. They were also asked whether there were any services not available in the area that would have enabled the person to remain out of residential care.

There were 50 people who required care 'then and now', and six who required it 'then but not now', who the assessors felt could have coped longer at home if the relevant services had been available. In Table 3.2 these 56 cases have been reclassified to group 3 - those judged to require residential care 'not then but now'. With the change the overall proportion assessed as not requiring residential care at the time of admission increases from 6.6 per cent in Table 3.1 to 17.2 per cent in Table 3.2. For those entering residential care from the community there is an increase from 11.3 per cent to 22.9 per cent.

Table 3.2
Need for residential care by source of admission(1)

Source of admission

Need for care:	From hospital		From other residential care		From the community		All admissions	
	N	%	N	%	N	%	N	%
1. Then and now	185	88.5	53	84.1	196	76.0	434	81.8
2. Then not now	1	0.5	1	1.6	3	1.2	5	0.9
3. Not then but now	23	11.0	7	11.1	41	15.9	71	13.4
4. Not then or now	-	-	2	3.2	18	7.0	20	3.8
Totals	209		63		258		530	100.0

$X^2 = 20.45$ $P < 0.01$

Notes:

1. 56 people were transferred from groups 1 or 2 in Table 3.1 to group 3 in Table 3.2 if they were considered able to cope longer at home providing relevant services had been available.

2. Same description of 4 groups as in Table 3.1.

If additional ordinary services such as sheltered housing or day care had been available at the time of admission the assessors believed that a further three or four per cent of the overall sample could have remained in the community. Added to the figure of 6.6 per cent who could have remained on the basis

3 9

of existing services this still represents only about one in ten residents admitted inappropriately. Even if more intensive services such as a full-time companion or a night sitting service had been available, residential care would still have been needed and appropriate in 83 per cent of cases.

Variations in need for residential care

There was some variation in the proportion of the sample not in need of residential care when admitted – that is groups 3 and 4 from Table 3.1. Table 3.3 indicates that the area with the lowest proportion of all admissions assessed as not in need was Devon (3.2 per cent) and the highest was Lothian (9.9 per cent). Residents in voluntary homes were more likely than those in private homes not to be in need of residential care. Those already in residence when assessed (retrospective cases) were no more likely to need residential care than those assessed in the process of entering (live cases). There were some differences in the proportion assessed as not needing residential care by each of the assessors. Thus, for example, in Sefton one of the assessors thought that 15 per cent of her cases were not in need of care when first admitted while her colleague considered that less than two per cent of her cases fell within the same category. Similar differences were also apparent in Lothian and Clwyd, the two other areas employing more than one assessor.

A proportion of this variation in assessors' judgements was certainly a function of the way their work was organised. In Lothian, for example, Assessor 2 had many more voluntary homes than either of her colleagues. Among her sample of homes were two large religious units both of which had undertaken extension and general upgrading of their accommodation. As a result both homes were able to offer a significant number of additional places to people whose level of need would not have previously ensured them a place. Likewise, variations between the two Sefton assessors may be partly explained by the fact that one saw nearly all the men in the sample, and a large proportion of residents in voluntary homes.

Those under 75 were less likely than those aged 75 and over to be considered in need of residential care and men living in residential homes were less likely than women to be considered in need of that type of care. There was some interaction between the different factors: for example 17 per cent of men aged under 75 and admitted to voluntary homes from the community were not in need of care.

Table 3.3
Proportion not in need of residential care
at time of admission (All admissions)

All admissions (N=530)

	Total	Not in need of residential care at admission	x^2
All	530	6.6	
Lothian	152	9.9	
Devon	156	3.2	7.3 NS
Sefton	112	8.9	
Clwyd	110	4.5	
In Private homes	378	4.5	8.3**
In Voluntary homes	152	11.8	
Retrospective	464	7.1	1.0 NS
Live	66	3.0	
Assessor: Lothian 1	39	10.3	
2	35	20.0	
3	78	5.1	
Devon	156	3.2	
Sefton 1	60	15.0	
2	52	1.9	25.1**
Clwyd 1	54	7.4	
2	56	1.8	
Age: Under 75	78	12.8	
75 or more	452	5.5	4.6*
Men residents	118	11.0	
Women residents	412	5.3	3.9*

Key: NS= Not significant; **= P<0.01; *= P<0.5

There were 182 homes included in the assessment study. Of
these, 155 had no one in the study not in need of residential
care. However there were five homes with more than one person
in the sample not in need. Three of these had two, one had
three and one had six. The home with six people assessed as
not in need of residential care was run by a religious order
and encouraged early entry. It had 15 residents in our sample.
One of the homes had two out of three residents in the sample
assessed as not in need. This home was run by a charity and

was described by the assessor as like a "5 Star Hotel with many residents fit and able". Apart from these two there appeared to be no special reason for the concentration of cases either in the homes or in the social workers who made the assessments in the homes.

Table 3.4 takes the analysis a stage further and presents the results in Column A for those elderly entering homes from the community who were judged by assessors not to be in need of care at the time of admission on the basis of existing services. Column B takes into account those who could have remained in the community longer had relevant services been available. The table shows that for every group the proportion not in need of care increases from those given in Table 3.3.

Table 3.4
Proportion not in need of residential care at time of admission (Admission from community)

Admission from community (N=258)

	Total	A Not in need of residential care at admission		B Not in need of residential care at admission	
	N	%	x^2	%	x^2
All	258	11.3		23.0	
Lothian	97	14.4		35.1	
Devon	74	5.4	4.2 NS	16.2	13.9**
Sefton	47	14.9		19.1	
Clwyd	40	10.3		10.3	
In Private homes	154	7.8		17.0	
In Voluntary homes	104	16.3	3.7 NS	31.7	6.8**
Retrospective	226	11.9		23.5	
Live	32	6.5	0.4 NS	19.4	0.8 NS
Assessor:					
Lothian 1	22	13.6		18.2	
2	28	25.0		60.7	
3	47	8.5		27.7	
Devon	74	5.4	14.2*	16.2	34.1**
Sefton 1	28	21.4		28.6	
2	19	5.3		5.3	
Clwyd 1	25	16.0		16.0	
2	15	-		-	
Age:					
Under 75	34	23.5		32.4	
75 or more	224	9.4	4.5*	21.5	1.4NS
Men residents	56	21.4		28.6	
Women residents	202	8.5	6.1*	21.4	0.9NS

Key: NS= Not significant; **= P<0.01; *P<0.05

Levels of dependency

Assessment, as recognised by the Joint Working Party, 'is not a precise or definitive process' (DHSS 1985, para. 3.7) – it rests on a judgement. How these judgements are made varies considerably. It has been shown, for example, that assessment is frequently undertaken by unqualified staff (Stapleton, 1977). Another investigation of local authority care in the Greater London area also highlighted considerable variations in the criteria and related procedures for admission (Neill, 1982). Compounding these problems has been a general uncertainty about the nature and purpose of assessment. A lack of clarity over some of the most commonly used concepts has also bedevilled attempts to derive valid and reliable measures of dependency and need. Although a number of well developed instruments for determining the physical and mental abilities of elderly people are available, such as the Modified Crighton Royal (MCR) Scale and the Clifton Assessment Procedures for the Elderly (COPE), they seldom form a component of local authority assessment.

The four areas in the present study were not using as part of their normal assessment any of the recognised scales of dependency. However, their social workers were making judgements about mobility, incontinence, memory and other important areas of dependency. In order to achieve consistency, so that we could compare like with like, it was decided to employ a standardised scale of dependency in the study. The MCR Scale was chosen because it was a well validated and widely used instrument. High levels of reliability and validity for the scale, especially high correlations between different raters, are reported (Charlesworth and Wilkin, 1982). Detailed notes, with examples of behaviour fitting the different categories, are also available for completing the scale. The MCR Scale contains ten items, five measuring physical capacity and five mental capacity. In addition to the separate scores for the ten individual items the scale also yields an overall score for all items, and sub-scores for physical capacity and mental capacity based on the relevant items for those dimensions.

For our purposes the scale also offered opportunities for comparison with other recent studies. Four in particular have employed the MCR Scale. Researchers at the Centre for Environmental and Social Studies in Ageing (CESSA) used the scale in their national study of 100 public sector residential homes (Willcocks, et al, 1982). Researchers at CESSA used it again in 1985 when studying private residential care in Norfolk (Weaver, et al, 1985). The Department of the Environment, in co-operation with DHSS, also used the scale in their study of

Table 3.5
MCR dependency scores of residents in independent and LA homes in five recent studies

| | INDEPENDENT HOMES | | | LOCAL AUTHORITY HOMES | | |
STUDY:	CESSA[1] (n=178) %	Devon[2] (n=392) %	York[3] (n=530) %	CESSA[4] (n=1000) %	Devon[2] (n=427) %	DoE[5] (n=999) %
Physical dependency						
Mobility						
0. Fully ambulant including stairs	40	48	36	34	34	38
1. Usually independent	15	15	21	21	19	22
2. Walks with supervision	14	11	10	9	7	6
3. Walks with aids or under care	17	22	26	26	31	27
4. Bedfast or chairfast	14	4	7	10	9	7
Dressing						
0. Correct	55	52	52	52	44	65
1. Imperfect but adequate	13	15	10	16	17	15
2. Adequate with minimum of supervision	9	12	15	13	12	11
3. Inadequate unless continually supervised	12	9	15	10	15	5
4. Unable to dress	11	12	8	9	14	4
Feeding						
0. Correct	80	76	80	79	77	88
1. Adequate with minimum of supervision	11	20	14	16	18	9
2. Inadequate unless continually supervised	6	2	5	3	2	2
3. Requires feeding	3	2	2	2	3	1
Bathing						
0. Washes and bathes without assistance	17	24	11	9	6	13
1. Minimal supervision with bathing	20	9	18	35	5	42
2. Close supervision with bathing	32	30	43	26	38	26
3. Inadequate unless continually supervised	10	17	18	7	26	5
4. Requires washing	21	21	10	23	25	14
Continence						
0. Full control	59	66	60	57	62	70
1. Occasional accidents	22	20	19	27	15	21
2. Continent by day regular toileting	5	3	7	5	5	3
3. Urinary incontinence	6	7	7	5	8	3
4. Regular or frequent double incontinence	8	4	7	6	10	2

Table 3.5 (Continued)

STUDY:	INDEPENDENT HOMES			LOCAL AUTHORITY HOMES		
	CESSA[1] (n=178) %	Devon[2] (n=392) %	York[3] (n=530) %	CESSA[4] (n=1000) %	Devon[2] (n=427) %	DoE[5] (n=999) %
Mental dependency						
Memory						
0. Complete	44	54	40	36	44	47
1. Occasionally forgetful	28	23	25	33	23	37
2. Short-term loss	14	10	20	10	11	8
3. Short- and long-term loss	14	13	14	21	22	8
Orientation						
0. Complete	66	66	52	46	51	60
1. Oriented in home	15	17	29	20	22	21
2. Misidentifies people	4	6	4	17	9	13
3. Cannot find way	5	4	8	7	6	4
4. Completely lost	10	7	7	10	12	2
Communication						
0. Always clear	58	63	57	45	47	60
1. Holds simple conversation	32	27	25	40	36	36
2. Simple conversation but does not indicate needs	3	5	11	4	7	1
3. Retains some expression	4	3	2	6	5	1
4. No effective contact	4	3	2	6	5	1
Co-operation						
0. Actively co-operative	76	71	65	47	59	59
1. Passively co-operative	17	20	19	28	25	26
2. Requires frequent encouragement	5	6	11	16	10	11
3. Rejects assistance	2	1	4	4	3	2
4. Completely resistive or withdrawn	–	2	1	5	3	1
Restlessness						
0. None	78	75	64	52	69	64
1. Intermittent	17	18	25	34	20	29
2. Persistent by day OR night	2	4	6	4	6	3
3. Persistent by day AND night	1	3	4	5	4	3
4. Constant	2	1	1	5	1	1

Refs:

1. Weaver, et al (1985)
2. Tibbenham (1985)
3. The present study
4. Willcocks, et al (1982)
5. Tinker (1984)

how a number of initiatives had enabled a sample of elderly people to remain in the community (Tinker, 1985). Of particular relevance to the present study was the comparative investigation by Devon Social Services Department of elderly residents in private and local authority care in the county (Tibbenham, 1985). The main focus of the study was the levels of dependency among residents in the two sectors, as measured by the MCR Scale. Table 3.5 presents the percentage distribution of results within the ten items of the scale for the various studies including the present study.

Table 3.5 above compared the MCR dependency scores for residents assessed in the present study with those obtained by other researchers. It is difficult to draw firm conclusions because the various studies were undertaken at different times, in different parts of the country and with the assessments made by different groups of people, not always social workers. However, in general, our sample drawn from private and voluntary homes tended to be slightly less independent than residents in similar homes in other studies.

Table 3.6 presents the results for the total score for each of the areas in the present study. Rather than presenting the whole range of scores we have adopted the method used by Tibbenham (1985) of collapsing these into three bands. The first, for those scoring 0 or only 1, represents fully independent/minimally dependent. The second, for those scoring between 2 and 10, covers the moderately dependent. The third, for those scoring 11 and more, the highly dependent.

The most notable feature of Table 3.6 is the position of Lothian, where significantly more elderly residents than in the other three areas were judged to be independent or only mildly dependent. In addition, there is little correspondence between the results for Devon in this study and the results from the County Council's own study of dependency in private homes in 1985 (Tibbenham, 1985). The major difference in approach was that our assessments were based on a social worker's face-to-face contact with the elderly person, whereas in the 1985 Devon study a research officer based his ratings on the proprietor's knowledge of the resident. This is not to discount, of course, the possibility that the two samples were drawn from very different populations, or that inter-rater reliability was very poor.

Table 3.6
MCR total score by area

Areas

Overall levels of dependency	Lothian	Devon	Sefton	Clwyd	All areas	Devon 1985 study
	%	%	%	%	%	%
Fully independent/mildly dependent Score 0, 1	19.2	2.6	8.2	2.5	8.9	18.1
Moderately dependent Score 2–10	59.6	52.9	50.9	48.1	53.7	52.3
Highly dependent Score 11 and over	21.3	44.5	40.9	49.4	37.4	29.6
Totals	100.0	100.0	100.0	100.0	100.0	100.0

$X^2 = 46.39$ $P < 0.0001$

Relating the total score to two other important independent variables also yielded significant results as Table 3.7 shows. Not surprisingly age was significantly related to dependence – the older the person, the greater their level of dependency. An even more significant relationship existed between dependency and the 'source of admission' to residential care. It was found that elderly people admitted to residential care from the community were less dependent than those admitted from hospital or other residential care. Table 3.7 also indicates the 'source of admission' was significantly related to levels of physical dependency but not mental dependency.

Table 3.7
MCR sub-scores and source of admission

Sources of admission

Physical levels of dependency	From hospital	From other residential care	From the community	All admissions
	%	%	%	%
Fully independent Score 0	1.9	4.8	13.0	7.6
Moderately dependent Score 1-9	72.5	76.2	72.8	73.1
Highly dependent Score 10 and over	25.6	19.0	14.2	19.3
Mental levels of dependency				
Fully independent Score 0	22.3	16.7	30.5	25.6
Moderately dependent Score 1-9	64.0	65.0	58.4	61.4
Highly dependent Score 10 and over	13.7	18.3	11.1	13.0
Totals	100.0	100.0	100.0	100.0

X^2 (Physical)= 26.88   P<0.0001 X^2 (Mental)= 7.66   NS

Table 3.8 presents the MCR sub-scores for physical and mental dependency in terms of the four categories of need. Not unexpectedly, in the light of previous results, the table indicates a highly significant relationship between levels of physical and mental dependency and need for residential care.

Table 3.8
MCR sub-scores and need for residential care

Physical levels of dependency	Then and now %	Then not now %	Not then but now %	Not then or now %	All %
Fully independent Score 0	5.2	18.2	26.7	45.0	7.6
Moderately dependent Score 1-9	73.8	72.7	73.3	55.0	73.1
Highly dependent Score 10 and over	20.9	9.1	—	—	19.3
Mental levels of dependency					
Fully independent Score 0	23.1	18.2	50.0	73.7	25.6
Moderately dependent Score 1-9	62.7	81.8	50.0	26.3	61.4
Highly dependent Score 10 and over	14.2	—	—	—	13.0
Totals	100.0	100.0	100.0	100.0	100.0

X^2(Physical)= 57.86 P<0.0001 X^2(Mental)= 32.16 P<0.0001

Reasons for admission

The assessor's opinion on the main reasons for admission are
given in Table 3.9. For those assessed as in need of care when
first admitted (groups 1 & 2) the most frequently mentioned set
of reasons for admission was that the person was no longer able
to cope by themselves, was at risk of depression or confusion,
was at risk of falling or fainting or had limited mobility due
to physical disablement or incapacity. The next most common
set of reasons for admission was that carers were no longer
able to cope. Less common reasons included unsatisfactory
accommodation, terminated leases and the death of a spouse or
other significant person. Table 3.10 provides an indication of
the relative importance of the reasons for admission of those
assessed as in need 'then and now'.

Table 3.9
The main reason for admission

	Groups 1 & 2 In need of residential care N=487 %	Groups 2 & 3 Not in need of residential care N=35 %
Person unable to care for themselves or cope alone any more	26.6	22.9
Principal informal carer not able to cope any longer	15.4	8.6
Person at risk because of depression/ confusion	14.5	-
Limited mobility	6.0	-
Person expressed desire for security and companionship	4.9	22.9
Person at risk of fainting or falls	4.3	-
Family no longer able to cope	4.3	-
Person needs 24 hour care	3.1	-
Lease on house terminated/home no longer available	2.9	17.0
Accommodation at home unsatisfactory	2.7	14.3
Person living alone and socially isolated	2.5	2.9
Death of spouse/other significant person	2.5	-
Indications of self-neglect	2.5	-
Hospital bed needed	2.3	-
Other reason	5.5	11.4
Totals	100.0	100.0

Table 3.10
Reasons for admission (Those in need 'then and now')

	A major reason %	A minor reason %	Not a reason %	DK %
Principal informal carer(s) not able to cope any longer	38.2	7.7	52.8	1.3
Person unable to care for themselves any more	84.8	8.5	6.4	0.2
Hospital bed no longer available/needed	23.6	10.3	63.8	2.3
Limited mobility due to physical disablement or incapacity	56.2	14.8	28.6	0.4
Person at risk because of fainting and/or falls	40.5	14.8	43.0	1.7
Person lived alone and socially isolated	33.3	12.3	53.1	1.3
Person expressed strong desire for security and companionship of residential home	26.3	14.2	54.8	4.8
Unsatisfactory accommodation/physical environment at home not suited for self-care	24.0	12.1	61.5	2.5
Indications of self-neglect	25.7	9.0	62.0	3.3
Person at risk because of depression and/or confusion	41.9	10.6	45.8	1.7
Indications of other forms of disturbed behaviour	15.8	3.2	64.1	16.8

For those who were admitted and not considered in need of
residential care the reasons for their admission had less to do
with their capacity for self care and the burden on carers than
their own wish for companionship and security, unsuitability of

their accommodation and the unavailability of sheltered accommodation.

Housing was a dominant factor associated with unnecessary admission to care. This is shown in Table 3.9 but perhaps more tellingly in the pen pictures in Annex 1. The majority of unnecessary admissions would have been more suitably catered for in supervised sheltered accommodation. It is the scarcity of that accommodation, particularly in the vicinity of supporting relatives, that led to a decision to enter residential care. Homelessness was also a factor - a number of the cases of unnecessary admissions were made homeless (not necessarily maliciously) through the actions of friends, landladies or relatives.

There were 31 cases (groups 2 and 4) who were still considered able to cope outside with appropriate accommodation and support services and again supervised sheltered accommodation was a dominant requirement. Nineteen could have coped in their own homes (and of these one was admitted from sheltered accommodation) and of the rest 11 would have required sheltered accommodation and one a resident carer placement.

Services

Table 3.11 provides a summary of the services being received before admission. In general a higher proportion of those in need of residential care had been receiving services before their admission. Thus for example half were receiving a home help, 45 per cent social work support, 28 per cent meals-on-wheels and 21 per cent warden served accommodation.

Those not in need of residential care when they were admitted were in general less likely to be receiving services - thus only a quarter were receiving home helps, seven per cent meals-on-wheels and 20 per cent social work support. Interestingly the only major service more likely to be being received by those not in need of residential care was sheltered housing and this may be an indication that being in sheltered housing is a reason for not being considered in need of residential care, a means of preventing it or that people in sheltered housing are at risk of being moved into care unnecessarily. In order to see whether more recent admissions were more likely to be receiving services the same table compares the results on the basis of whether the assessment was retrospective or live. In general those assessed live were more likely to be receiving services.

Table 3.11
Services received before admission (all admissions N=530)

	Groups 1&2 In need of residential care	Groups 3&4 Not in need of residential care	Retro- spective assessments	Live assessments
	N=495 %	N=35 %	N=464 %	N=66 %
Community nurse	32.9	3.4	30.8	33.3
Chiropody	24.8	27.6	23.9	32.8
Physiotherapy	17.0	10.3	15.3	26.8
Health visitor	12.5	10.3	11.4	20.0
Social worker	45.0	20.0	41.9	55.4
Home help	51.1	26.7	48.5	57.6
Laundry	1.8	–	1.7	1.8
Incontinence services	4.5	–	4.5	1.8
Meals-on-wheels	27.6	7.1	25.7	31.6
Luncheon club	7.0	25.0	8.0	8.9
Day care	17.9	14.3	17.3	20.8
Sheltered housing	20.9	27.6	20.9	24.1
Alarm system	24.2	34.5	23.4	35.7
Short stay care	14.9	3.3	13.2	21.4

In Table 3.12 we see that those not in need of residential care were much more likely to have had an unmet need for services before admission and in a number of cases social workers commented that services that were available including psychiatric treatment, night care and, most common, sheltered

Table 3.12
Not receiving services and in need of them
before admission (all admissions N=530)

	Groups 1&2 In need of residential care N=495 %	Groups 3&4 Not in need of residential N=35 %	Retro- spective assessments N=464 %	Live assessments N=66 %
Community nurse	7.3	10.3	7.3	8.8
Chiropody	8.0	-	8.1	3.4
Physiotherapy	3.9	-	3.6	3.6
Health visitor	8.7	13.8	9.4	5.5
Social worker	19.8	43.3	22.0	16.1
Home help	13.2	33.3	15.5	6.8
Laundry	17.2	10.3	17.8	8.8
Incontinence services	4.2	-	4.0	3.5
Meals-on-wheels	18.2	25.0	19.4	12.3
Luncheon club	14.7	7.1	14.7	14.7
Day care	30.3	21.4	31.0	20.8
Sheltered housing	17.3	34.5	18.4	19.0
Alarm system	13.7	20.7	14.1	14.3
Short stay care	18.4	23.3	19.4	14.3

housing could have prevented admission to care. Live admissions were less likely to have an unmet need for a number of the services including home helps, day care, meals-on-wheels and social work support.

As we have seen the assessors considered that 93 per cent of the overall sample were in need of residential care when first admitted. However, as mentioned earlier, they also considered that 56 of these cases (11.3 per cent) could have remained at home if other services had been available. The services required by most of these cases were invariably intensive such as extra care sheltered housing, psycho-geriatric day care, night sitting services, full day care with some night support, a full-time companion. However in 20 cases the services required were of a more normal nature - suitable housing near a relative, a local day centre, adequate heating, intensive home help services, convalescent facilities and most common of all (in 14 of the 20 cases) warden supervised sheltered housing. It appears that the assessors in Lothian and Sefton were particularly likely to assess a person in need of residential care because of the absence or shortage of sheltered accommodation.

It is arguable whether these 20 cases (3.8 per cent of the whole sample) should be added to those found not in need of residential care at the time of admission. They appear to be in need of care only because appropriate accommodation and services were not available when and where they were needed. If they were included among those not in need of care then the proportion would increase to be 10.4 per cent of the whole sample and 19 per cent of those admitted from the community.

Process of admission

Table 3.13 compares those who were involved in initiating the move into residential care. For those in need of care relatives were most likely to be involved in initiating admission. For those in need of care the move to a residential home was most commonly initiated by the elderly person themselves or again a relative. While friends, neighbours and landlords were also important sources of referral for this group doctors and social workers were rarely involved.

Table 3.13
Person(s) initiating move into residential care

	Groups 1&2 In need of residential care N=495 %	Groups 3&4 Not in need of residential care N=35 %
General practitioner	31.7	5.7
Geriatrician/psychiatrist other hospital doctor/ hospital staff	27.7	-
Local area based social worker	17.2	2.9
Hospital based social worker	27.1	-
The elderly person (ie. self-referral)	29.3	65.7
Relatives	53.3	45.7
Friends/neighbours	4.6	17.1
Landlord	0.6	14.3
Warden - sheltered housing	1.4	-
Staff previous residential home	2.2	2.9
Staff present residential home	1.2	2.9
Clergy/church, etc.	0.8	5.7
Community nurse/health visitor	3.2	2.9
Other	1.4	2.9
Not known	0.2	-

Table 3.14
Person(s) involved in assessing need for residential
care prior to admission (all admissions N=530)

	Groups 1&2 In need of residential care N= 495 %	Groups 3&4 Not in need of residential care N= 35 %
General practitioner	44.2	31.4
Geriatrician/psychiatrist other hospital doctor/ hospital staff	35.2	2.9
Local area based social worker	21.0	2.9
Hospital based social worker	29.5	-
Other social services/work department personnel	3.0	2.9
Professional staff employed at the home	32.5	65.7
Professional staff employed by a voluntary organistion	2.2	2.9
Community nurse/health visitor	3.2	-
Proportion where doctor involved in assessment	69.3	34.3
Proportion where doctor or MSW involved in assessment	72.9	34.3
Proportion where social services/social work involvement	49.1	5.7
Proportion where doctor and social work involvement	38.4	2.9
Proportion where only home staff involved	4.6	34.3
Percentage assessed	77.2	71.4

Table 3.14 provides information on whether any assessment was carried out before admission. Of those in need of care on admission, multi-disciplinary assessments (in the sense that both a doctor and a social worker were involved) had been made in 38 per cent of cases. Personnel from the Social Services or Social Work Department were involved in assessment in 49 per cent of cases. In only five per cent of cases of those in need of care when admitted was the only assessment carried out by the home. In contrast those admitted who were not in need were much less likely to have had any independent assessment and where they had been assessed it was most likely to have been by the home or by their GP. Social work personnel assessed only six per cent and in 34 per cent the only assessment carried out was by staff in the home.

As we have already described, arrangements for multi-disciplinary assessment only existed in Lothian and for some cases in Sefton. This is reflected in the results in Table 3.15 which show that both these areas have the highest proportion where doctors and social workers were or might have been involved in assessment.

Table 3.15
Proportion assessed by doctors and social workers
(In need of care groups 1 & 2)

Involved in assessment	Lothian	Devon	Sefton	Clwyd	All
Doctors and social workers	40.9	33.1	53.9	27.6	38.4
Hospital social worker	24.8	20.5	47.1	31.4	29.5
Hospital social workers and other social workers	-	2.0	10.8	1.0	3.0

In the course of their inquiries the social work assessors had found that at the time of admission there had not always been unanimity about the need for care among the various participants in the referral. For example, in 21 per cent of the cases judged later by the assessors as not in need of care, and in 54 per cent of those judged in need of care, there had originally existed differences in opinion. Disputes were most common between the residents and their relatives and seemed to arise where the relatives felt guilt about a situation breaking down, or where they had come to a decision to put the elderly person into care and had arranged an admission without counsulting them. Disputes also arose between the elderly person and doctors or social workers when the elderly person did not feel ready to move out of their own home and felt 'pushed into' residential care.

The assessors agreed that 'reluctance' and 'conflict' could be confused and assessments should look for both and handle them differently. Unless very demented the elderly person should have the final decision where possible - conflict about the move will make it much more difficult for them to 'settle'. Once wrongly placed it is very difficult, if not impossible, for the elderly person to return to the community because they have usually given up their home and disposed of their furniture.

4 The process of assessment

So far we have concentrated on various items relating to the outcome of the assessment undertaken by the social work assessors for the research. In this chapter we describe how they carried out the assessment.

Factors taken into account

Assessors were asked which aspects of dependency they took into account in assessing the need for residential care and in almost all the cases they claimed to have taken account of all of them. The majority of the assessors also said that in making their judgements they took account of the availability of services in the area, the housing accommodation the person had been occupying and the availability and circumstances of carers.

Sources of information

These varied, as might be expected, with whether the person was already resident in the home when assessed or in the process of being admitted. Table 4.1 summarises the main results. For those already in homes the home owner was the most important source of information for the assessment, followed closely by the elderly people themselves, social workers and relatives.

Table 4.1
Importance of sources of information

	Retrospective assessments %	Live assessments %
Elderly person		
Very important	67	73
Quite important	21	15
Not important	6	2
Not consulted	6	11
Relatives		
Very important	31	38
Quite important	4	5
Not important	1	–
Not consulted	65	57
Home owner		
Very important	79	71
Quite important	20	25
Not important	–	3
Not consulted	–	2
GP		
Very important	5	10
Quite important	2	12
Not important	1	3
Not consulted	92	75
Area based social worker (those who had had one)		
Very important	47	85
Quite important	7	5
Not important	1	–
Not consulted	45	10
Hospital based social worker (those admitted from hospital)		
Very important	47	88
Quite important	4	4
Not important	4	–
Not consulted	45	8
Others who were very or quite important		
Spouse (those with)	61	50
Friends	3	10
Hospital doctor (admitted from hospital)	15	10
Health visitor (those who had one)	12	20
Community nurse (those who had one)	10	–
Medical records	17	33
Others not consulted		
Spouse (those with)	32	50
Friends	97	91
Hospital doctor (admitted from hospital)	84	90
Health visitor (those who had had one)	88	80
Community nurse (those who had had one)	89	100
Medical records	83	65

In the case of those in the process of entering the elderly person and the home owner were still very important but in addition relatives, the GP, medical records and social workers were more likely to be consulted.

Among potential sources of information that were least likely to be consulted were health service personnel - health visitors, community nurses and hospital doctors (though in the latter case a hospital based social worker could have consulted the doctor).

Time taken in the assessment

The assessors were asked to record how long it took to carry out the assessment of each person excluding any time that they spent completing the research questionnaire. The results are summarised in Table 4.2. On average assessments took about two and a half hours - about 40 minutes travelling, about an hour interviewing and half an hour writing up. The time spent on assessment of those in the process of entry was not significantly different from the time spent on those already in homes. The assessor's travel time was slightly shorter and their use of the telephone slightly longer.

The average time taken on assessment hides considerable variations - thus for example travel time varied from nil to three and a half hours and interviews with the home owners where they took place lasted up to two hours. In all, assessments varied from 30 minutes to five and three quarter hours. There was some variation between the areas. Among those already in homes, Lothian assessments took about half an hour less than Sefton assessments on average. Among the assessors the time varied between 2 hours for one of the Lothian assessors to 3 hours for one of the Sefton assessors but these variations may well be a function of how cases were distributed between assessors as much as the practices of the assessors. There was a rather wider range of variation among those in the process of entry - though the numbers are small.

Time span of assessment

As well as the time involved in carrying out assessments, one of the factors to be considered is how quickly they can be carried out. In order to provide some indication of this, assessors were asked how many working days the assessments took, ie. how many days elapsed from making the initial arrangement to completing the written assessment. The results are summarised in Table 4.3. Overall it took seven and a half days for those already in homes and six and a half days for those in the process of admission.

Table 4.2
Time taken in assessment

	Retrospective assessments Mean (minutes) N= 464		Live assessments Mean (minutes) N= 66	
Preparation and initial arrangements	9		9	
Telephone calls	12		14	
Travel	41		34	
Interviewing person/appointee	28		32	
Interviewing manager	24		20	
Interviewing third parties	6		5	
Consulting records	6		8	
Writing up	31		37	
Other (waiting time, thinking, observation)	1		0	
Totals	156		161	NS
	Mean (mins)	N	Mean (mins)	N
Lothian	134	128	166	24
Devon	158	144	119	12
Sefton	169	96	176	16
Clwyd	171	96	170	14
Assessor:				
Lothian 1	133	32	172	7
2	130	29	160	6
3	137	67	164	11
Devon	158	144	119	12
Sefton 1	157	53	175	7
2	184	43	177	9
Clwyd 1	176	48	206	6
2	166	48	143	8
In need of residential care:				
Then and now	157	420	160	64
Then not now	147	11	-	-
Not then but now	154	15	-	-
Not then or now	152	18	210	2

Table 4.3
Time (days) elapsed in making the assessment

	Retrospective assessments Mean	N	Live assessments Mean	N
In need of residential care				
Then and now	7.8	418	6.4	62
Then not now	5.4	11	-	-
Not then but now	6.9	15	-	-
Not then not now	6.8	18	3.0	1
Lothian	4.2	128	5.3	22
Devon	10.0	144	6.4	12
Sefton	8.3	95	7.9	16
Clwyd	8.2	95	6.1	13
Assessor:				
Lothian 1	6.9	32	5.1	7
2	4.8	29	6.2	6
3	2.7	67	4.8	9
Devon	10.0	144	6.4	12
Sefton 1	6.7	53	5.9	7
2	10.2	42	9.4	9
Clwyd 1	9.8	48	7.2	5
2	6.5	47	5.4	8
All	7.6	462	6.3	63 NS
Missing cases=	2		3	

We are not certain that this represents a very good indication of how long it would take in the real world. The assessors in our project were working with a large pile of cases on their desks. Even the assessments of people entering during the project had to compete for attention with other cases. Furthermore, some of the assessors were working part-time. The time taken will have depended on how the assessors arranged their work and it is noticeable in that context that one of the Lothian assessors completed her cases in two and a half days on average while one of the Sefton assessors, took over ten days. When we spoke to the assessors about this finding those in Lothian told us they had calculated the time from the first face to face contact to the completion of the write-up. However, assessors in the other areas had include

the period between writing or telephoning for an appointment
and visiting the home. Thus, a figure of between six and seven
days is a slight underestimate of the time elapsed in making
the assessment.

Problems in making the assessment

The assessors said that they had had problems making the
assessment in about a third of the cases, though there were
rather fewer problems among the live assessments. The problems
they experienced are summarised in Table 4.4. The most common
were the mental confusion of the elderly person in about 40 per
cent of the retrospective assessments, relatives unavailable
for interview in 18 per cent, lack of information in 18 per
cent and miscellaneous delays in 16 per cent.

One of the reasons for adequate information not being
available in the homes related. to movements of residents
between homes, or changes of management. Several home
owners/managers remarked that they would welcome the idea of a
standardised assessment/social history form, a copy of which
could be retained at the home and which would be sent on to the
new home if a resident moved.

Table 4.4
Problems experienced in carrying out the assessment

	Retrospective assessments N=464 %	Live assessments N=66 %
Mental confusion	38.7	40.0
Relatives not available	18.2	25.0
Lack of information	17.7	15.0
Miscellaneous delays	16.0	5.0
Problems of access/ confidentiality	13.8	5.0
Resident from outside area	6.6	20.0
Resident uncooperative	6.1	5.0
Confused information/ inappropriate referral or placement	4.4	15.0
Mentioning problems (N)	181	20
Percentage (%)	39.0	30.3

The declaration

If assessment by social service/social work departments is introduced there may need to be a certificate of need or eligibility which can be completed by the assessor and sent to DHSS by the claimant with their claim for board and lodging allowance. This is rather on the model of the family doctor's sick note. As part of the study we included at the suggestion of DHSS the following mock Recommendation for Residential Care:

> On the basis of my enquiries it is my professional judgement that **NAME OF PERSON** is/is not* in need of residential care of the type provided at **NAME OF HOME**. His/her need for such care should be reviewed in **XX** months.

Assessors had no difficulty in completing the first part of this recommendation.

Need for review

Assessors found it more difficult to recommend when a review should take place. Table 4.5 summarises the results. In about a quarter of cases no recommendation for review was made. In five per cent it was just left blank and this may have been an oversight in completing the questionnaire. In 19 per cent of cases the recommendation had been crossed out and in one per cent the assessors had overwritten "impossible to say". The reasons given by assessors for not making a review or deleting the recommendation varied. Many found it difficult to make a judgement. In some cases the assessor was satisfied that the person was well placed and a review was therefore unnecessary. In other cases the assessor expected the person to die or deteriorate and no further assessment would be required except admission to hospital. There was also confusion about what the purpose of the review was. Was it to reconsider the need for residential care; to review the appropriateness of the placement in that type of home; to review the category of care within the home; or all three? Clearly the mock certificate is unsatisfactorily ambiguous and needs to be revised.

Table 4.5
Recommendations for review

In	%
1 month	2.0
2 months	0.8
3 months	19.8
6 months	36.7
12 months	32.4
15 months	0.3
18 months	0.8
24 months	7.3

Not able to make a recommendation   25% (N= 132)

	Mean months	(SD)	N
In need of residential care:			
Then and now	8.9	(5.7)	367
Then not now	5.4	(1.3)	5
Not then but now	5.6	(3.4)	12
Not then or now	5.2	(3.3)	14
Retrospective assessment	8.9	(5.6)	340
Live assessment	6.9	(5.8)	58
All	8.6	(5.7)	398

Where recommendations were made those in need of residential care had longer periods recommended before review than those not in need. Retrospective cases also had longer review periods on average than live assessments.

The assessors indicated that, ideally, reviews should be undertaken every three months during the first two years and every six months thereafter – unless there was little hope of improvement, in which case it should be every six months. In all cases it is important to involve the elderly person, their family and the care staff in the review. From a social work point of view it is not the need for care which should be reviewed but the suitability of the care at present provided.

5 The background of the residents

Admission date

Of those people who were already resident when the assessment began in September 1986 the average length of stay in that home was 16 months. The length ranged from less than a month to 19 years. The distribution of length in residence is given in Table 5.1.

Table 5.1
Length of stay in present residential care
home (Retrospective cases)

	N	%
Less than 1 month	2	0.4
1-3 months	66	14.2
4-6 months	77	16.6
7-9 months	77	16.6
10-12 months	55	11.9
13-18 months	71	15.3
19-24 months	60	12.9
More than 24 months	56	12.1
Totals	464	100.0

Admission from local area or away

One of the matters to be decided if assessment is introduced is what happens when people are admitted from outside the area.

Nearly a quarter of our sample were admitted from outside the social services area in which the home was situated. There was no evidence that those not in need of residential care were more likely to be admitted from outside the area. The distance from the previous home is summarised in Table 5.2.

Table 5.2
Those admitted from outside area

	Lothian %	Devon %	Sefton %	Clwyd %	All %
Admitted from outside area	13.2	22.4	50.0	13.6	23.8
Distance (miles)					
0-25	-	20.6	41.1	13.3	26.0
26-50	11.1	5.9	28.6	13.3	17.9
51-100	22.2	17.6	17.9	33.3	20.3
100+	66.7	55.9	10.7	40.0	35.0
Outside the UK	-	-	1.8	-	0.8
Totals	18	34	56	15	123

About 44 per cent had been admitted from within 50 miles of the residential home but 35 per cent had come from over 100 miles away. However the situation is very different in different areas. Sefton has by far the highest proportion admitted from outside the area - half - but most of these are admitted from within 50 miles - from Lancashire and Merseyside. About a quarter of Devon's admission came directly from outside the area but more than half of these are from over 100 miles away. Lothian has a very small proportion of incomers but most of those come from over 100 miles away. Similar to Lothian, Clwyd also has a small proportion of incomers, over three-quarters of whom came from over 50 miles away.

As well as those admitted to residential homes from outside the local authority area we were interested to discover what proportion of admissions from those within the area were long-standing residents and what proportion had retired to the area before admission. This information is summarised in Table 5.2.

Table 5.3
Those admitted from within area

	Lothian %	Devon %	Sefton %	Clwyd %	All %
Proportion admitted from area	86.8	77.6	50.0	86.4	76.2
Retired to area	15.9	39.8	24.5	23.9	26.1
Did not retire to area	84.1	60.2	75.5	76.1	73.9

X2= 18.9   P<0.001

	In need of care N=365 %	Not in need of care N=27 %
Retired to area	25.5	33.3
Did not retire to area	74.5	66.7

X2= 0.44 NS

Proportion living less than five years in area before admission

	%	N
Lothian	3.0	132
Devon	10.7	121
Sefton	-	56
Clwyd	3.2	95
Totals	5.0	404

Mean length of time in areas

	Years Mean	(SD)	N
Lothian	62.4	(27.8)	132
Devon	42.4	(30.5)	118
Sefton	46.5	(29.5)	53
Clwyd	42.5	(26.0)	90
All	49.7	(29.8)	395

F=13.5   P<0.001

Missing cases= 9

Overall 26 per cent of those admitted to the homes from the local area had moved to the area after retirement but again the proportion varied considerably from about 16 per cent in Lothian to 40 per cent in Devon. There is no evidence that those who retired into the area were more likely to have been admitted to residential homes without being in need. Only one in twenty of those who move to an area before entering residential care live in their own homes for less than five years and, on average, people admitted from their own area have lived there for nearly 50 years - Lothian had the most stable entrants - their residents had been there for over 60 years on average.

These results indicate that if assessment was introduced it would present rather different problems in different areas. An area like Devon with a high proportion of admission from areas some distance away would have to make greater use of assessors working as agents for them. Areas with a high proportion of retirees into the area who quickly move into residential care may also need to have some aspects of an assessment undertaken in the home area.

Known to social services

At the time of admission to the residential home there was known to be a live case file in the social services/social work department for 61 per cent of those admitted from the local area and 65 per cent of those admitted from hospital. In comparison, only 29 per cent of those admitted from outside the local area were known to have had a case file.

Table 5.4 shows that the existence of a live case file was associated with whether the person needed residential care. It was particularly striking that only two of the 20 cases not in need of residential care now or when admitted had a case file. The table also shows that the proportion with a case file varied from area to area with only 34 per cent of admissions in Sefton known to have one, compared with 64 per cent in Lothian and Devon. This result for Sefton is partly explained by the high proportion of admissions from outside their area.

Table 5.4
Proportion with a live case file available

	%	N
Admitted from area	61.1	401
Admitted from outside	28.6	126
Admitted from hospital	64.6	208
Admitted from community	50.4	256
Admitted from other		
residential care	30.2	63
In need of care:		
Then and now	55.5	481
Then not now	45.5	11
Not then but now	46.7	15
Not then or now	10.0	20
Lothian	63.8	152
Devon	64.1	156
Sefton	33.9	112
Clwyd	43.0	107
Totals	53.3	527
Missing cases=		3

Proportions with a live case file	Admitted from hospital	Admitted from community	Admitted from other residential care
Admitted from area	71.9	56.8	41.5
Admitted from outside	39.1	28.1	9.1

Supplementary benefit history

In a random sample drawn from the population aged over 80 we would expect only 26 per cent to be on SB (DHSS 1984). The proportion in this study on SB before admission to residential care, about 47 per cent, is far higher than one would expect even allowing for the age structure of the sample. Table 5.5 shows that the proportion of retrospective and live cases on SB before entry was similar. However, the proportion of live cases who came straight onto SB at entry is greater than the proportion of retrospective cases. Of those who were not on SB before they entered 71 per cent came onto SB as soon as they were admitted and a further 15 per cent were on SB within three months of entry. Our sample was supposed to be restricted to people who had been claiming supplementary benefit at their present address for one or at the most two years after entry and this explains why the majority of those who came onto supplementary benefit after entry had been on for quite short periods. There were 25 cases who found their way into the sample who had been on SB and in the existing home for more than two years. Seventeen of those were Devon cases that may have been included in the sample by the assessor. The rest were either selected in error by local offices at the initial sampling stage or the information elicited by assessors about this item is wrong.

Because of the nature of the sampling method it is not possible to draw firm conclusions about the likely balance of assessments between those in the process of entry and those already in care coming on to benefit. Nevertheless it is striking that such a large proportion of the sample were on SB before entry or came onto SB on entry. It looks from this that there will be a relatively small proportion of the population requiring assessment after entry when their resources had run out.

Table 5.5
Supplementary benefit history

	Retrospective assessments		Live assessments		All	
	N	%	N	%	N	%
On supplementary benefit before admission	196	46.2	27	50.0	223	46.7
Came onto supplementary benefit on entry	155	36.6	25	46.3	180	37.7
Came onto supplementary benefit						
1 month after entry	20	4.7	2	3.7	22	4.6
2-3 months after entry	13	3.1	–		13	2.7
4-6 months after entry	7	1.7	–		7	1.5
6-12 months after entry	9	2.1	–		9	1.9
1-2 years after entry	7	1.7	–		7	1.5
2 years plus	17	4.0	–		17	3.6
Totals	424	100.0	54	100.0	478	100.0
Missing cases=		40		12		

Only two per cent of the sample (9 cases) had had any break in their SB since entering residential homes. The reasons for this were either a spell in different accommodation, capital resources exceeding the limit or the sale of a house. Again this result may be partly a function of the nature of our sample – cases in homes and on benefit for less than two years. However the very low level of volatility in claiming is striking and quite unexpected.

Present status

Table 5.6 summarises the present category of supplementary benefit being received by the elderly person. Nearly three-quarters were categorised as elderly only and a further 15 per cent as very dependent elderly. This last percentage is rather high given that only 10 per cent of the sample were in receipt of attendance allowance at the higher rate, the criterion for the very dependent category. Part of the discrepancy can be explained by the fact that blind people have been identified separately. There are two qualifying conditions for the higher limit of £145 – receipt of attendance allowance at the higher rate or blindness. The blind also qualify for the blind addition.

Table 5.6
Present SB status of resident

	%	N
Elderly	73.4	384
Mentally handicapped	0.2	1
Mentally ill	7.1	37
Very dependent elderly	15.3	80
Disabled under pension age	1.1	6
Blind	2.3	12
Drug or alcohol dependent	0.6	3
Totals	100.0	523

Missing cases or not known because not yet in receipt   N= 7

Attendance/mobility allowance

Eighteen per cent of this sample were in receipt of attendance allowance – ten per cent at the higher rate and 1.7 per cent were receiving the mobility allowance.

Other sources of income

In addition to SB, retirement pension, and attendance and mobility allowances, Table 5.7 summarises what other sources of income were being received by residents. The most common was an occupational pension received by 18 per cent. Of course none of these sources of income made any difference to living standards as they would be being taken into account in assessing SB.

Table 5.7
Other sources of income

	%	N
War pension	1.7	9
Occupational pension	18.0	94
Widow's pension	1.0	4
Blind/Disability/Invalidity/ Sickness Benefit	2.1	2
Maintenance	0.6	3

Charges for the accommodation

Table 5.8 summarises the weekly charge being made for the accommodation. There is considerable variation in charges – from £45 to £185. However there is a clear bunching of charges at the SB limits. Thus a third of the sample are being charged £125 per week – the supplementary benefit limit for an elderly person living in a home registered to care for the elderly, and 17 per cent were being charged at £120 – the old limit. The mean charge is also almost £125 per week. The average charge is lowest in Clwyd and highest in Devon. The charges in private homes are on average higher than charges in voluntary homes.

Table 5.8
Weekly charge to the resident

	%	N
Less than £100	6.1	32
£100 – £119	12.0	63
£120	16.9	89
£121 – £124	2.7	14
£125	33.6	177
£126 – £129	0.9	5
£130	8.0	42
£131 – £139	4.4	23
£140	6.1	32
£140+	9.5	50
Totals	100.0	527

	Mean £	SD	N
Lothian	124	(14.1)	152
Devon	128	(18.2)	156
Sefton	126	(11.7)	111
Clwyd	121	(11.4)	108
Private	129	(11.9)	376
Voluntary	115	(16.1)	151
All	125	(14.8)	527

Table 5.9 shows the average charge being made for residents in different categories of care. Charges are highest for the mentally ill and the very dependent elderly.

Table 5.10 provides a distribution of the difference between the SB limit for the particular category of care and the charge being made by the home. The differences vary from between £95 less than the limit to £45 above the limit. Overall, 21 per cent of homes visited in the sample are charging more than the limit – 26.5 per cent of homes in the private sector but only 8 per cent of homes in the voluntary sector.

Table 5.9
Charge by category of care

	Mean £	SD	N
Elderly	123	(13.5)	381
Mentally handicapped	125	–	1
Mentally ill	132	(10.5)	37
Very dependent elderly	131	(19.4)	80
Disabled under pensionable age	128	(15.2)	6
Blind	127	(16.4)	12
Drug or alcohol dependent	123	(2.9)	3
All	125	(14.8)	520

Missing cases= 10

Table 5.10
Distribution of the difference between the SB limit and the weekly charge

	Private home		Voluntary home		All	
	N	%	N	%	N	%
£ less than the limit:						
95–31	5		10			
30–21	4		24			
20–16	23		4			
15–11	28		37			
10–6	16	37.7	6	71.9	246	47.3
5–1	65		24			
same as the limit:	134	35.8	30	20.5	164	31.5
£ more than the limit:						
1–5	31		2			
6–10	18		4			
11–15	9	26.5	1	7.5	110	21.2
16–20	14		2			
21–30	17		–			
31–45	10		2			
Totals	374	100.0	146	100.0	520	100.0

Missing cases= 10

Table 5.11 shows that the mean charge over the limit was £15.20 and it varied between £20.50 in Devon to £7.20 in Clwyd. As well as more private homes charging over the limit the amount by which they exceed the limit is slightly higher than voluntary homes. Lothian is interesting that it has a high proportion of residents in voluntary homes, and also a high proportion of its homes charging over the limit. This is because private homes in Lothian appear to have relatively high charges.

Table 5.11
Charge over the limit

	Mean £	SD	N	%over limits
Lothian	16.10	(8.8)	40	27.2
Devon	20.50	(12.0)	34	21.9
Sefton	10.30	(10.2)	24	21.6
Clwyd	7.20	(6.5)	12	11.2
Private	15.30	(10.7)	99	26.5
Voluntary	14.50	(13.5)	11	7.5
All	15.20	(10.9)	110	21.2

Topping up

As we have seen 21 per cent of the sample were paying more than the SB limit for their category of accommodation. How were they managing to meet the difference? Table 5.12 summarises the position for the 61 residents where information is given. The most common source of topping up was the personal allowance - more than a half of those needing topping up were using this source of income. Apart from this, contribution from relatives (35 per cent) and disregarded personal savings (24 per cent) were the most common forms of topping up help.

Those using their personal allowance had to top up their SB by an average of £12.60 - more than the personal allowance of £9.05, though less than the average topping up received from relatives, savings or charity.

Table 5.12
Topping up

Proportion with	%	Mean topping up £	N
Contribution from relatives	36.1	16.10	22
Contribution from a charity	8.2	25.20	5
From DHSS personal allowance	54.1	12.60	33
From personal savings	24.6	17.50	15
All		17.85	61

Missing cases= 49

Types of room

Over half (55 per cent) of the sample are living in single rooms and most of the rest are in double rooms. However, 5 per cent are in rooms with three or four beds. The average charge paid for different types of room does not vary.

Suitability of home

The social work assessors concluded that for those who required residential care now, the home they were in was suitable for all but three per cent (16 cases). The following settings were judged by the assessors to offer more appropriate forms of care for the 16 cases - a nursing home (6 cases), a hospital (4 cases) and another residential home offering a different category of care (6 cases).

6 Discussion of the assessment study

Is it worth it?

The proportion of elderly people in private and voluntary homes for the elderly who were found not to be in need of such care at the time of admission was very small. As few as 6.6 per cent if account is taken of existing services, about 10 per cent if ordinary domiciliary services or sheltered housing had been available, and no more than 17.2 per cent if alternative, more intensive relevant services had also been available.

Given the nature of the study and particularly the fact that most of the assessments of need for care were made retrospectively with limited access to pertinent information there are obviously grounds for being cautious about the validity of this finding. However it is reassuring that those assessed 'live' were found to be no less in need of residential care. These judgements are often difficult and complex even in a real situation requiring as they do the weighing up of the elderly person's needs and preferences; those of carers; and the effectiveness of the support likely to be available from the statutory and voluntary sectors. They will rarely ever be cut and dried. The social workers <u>were</u> able to make judgements about need which they were prepared to uphold. They did identify people not in need of residential care and they did identify more appropriate forms of care.

The proportion found not to be in need of care was very
small. However, there is evidence of some unnecessary and
premature admission to residential homes. In some of these
cases it is because of the under-utilisation of and ignorance
about the alternatives available. In other cases it is because
services or facilities were not available or not enough of them
were available - particularly warden supported sheltered
housing. Some of those who entered homes unnecessarily went in
willingly and of their own volition - they often felt they
would eventually need care and wanted to "settle in" before a
crisis. Others who entered homes unnecessarily went in against
their will advised and assisted by relatives with a vested
interest, even if only for their own peace of mind. In the
vast majority of these cases of unnecessary admission there had
been no dispassionate assessment of need.

Yet given the small numbers identified as not in need of
residential care in this study is it worth screening all
prospective entrants to independent homes? One factor to weigh
up is the costs and savings that would be involved.
Unfortunately that is no simple matter and this study can only
help point to the elements that would need to be taken into
account in such a calculation.

(1) Benefits: Each supplementary pensioner in the community
costs about £60 a week in pension (including contributory and
supplementary pension) plus housing benefit. In a number of
cases attendance allowance, invalid care allowance or domestic
assistance addition will also be received. In residential care
each elderly person can be assessed to cost, say, £135 a week
(the limit for elderly people plus the personal expenses
allowance). Clearly for each person deterred from entering
residential care from the community there would be savings to
the social security budget. However, an important
consideration is that supplementary benefit, housing benefit,
attendance allowance and invalid care allowance may be payable
to a person in their own home. In such cases the difference
between the benefit payable in a residential care home and in a
person's own home may be very small. Any savings to the social
security budget would also need to be set against the costs of
assessment, the costs of additional support in the community
from health and social services and the opportunity costs to
carers.

(2) The costs of alternative care: The economic case for
assessment will depend crucially on how much it would cost to
maintain those not in need of care in the community. This
study did not attempt to assess the costs of alternative
packages of care. However, the Kent Community Care scheme

(Davies and Challis, 1986) has demonstrated that it is possible to sustain elderly people at high risk in the community at two thirds of the institutional cost, given imaginative case management with devolved budgeting systems. The introduction of assessment might itself act as a catalyst in enabling local agencies to plan more coherent services for elderly people, enabling many more of them to stay in the community for longer periods of time. A dynamic situation of this sort is another reason why the probable cost-effectiveness of assessment is difficult to forecast.

(3) The costs of assessment: Our assessments took from two and a half to three hours each and the DHSS made a contribution towards the local authorities' costs. It is not possible to extrapolate from the costs of assessing care needs in this study to the costs of assessment in the real world. We were unable to measure the true costs to the authorities involved in carrying out this pilot scheme but it was almost certainly more than the general contribution made by DHSS to the research as a whole.

Because of practical constraints, our assessments were not the same as the authorities' own assessments. The latter almost certainly take longer and cost more - particularly where, as in Lothian, a medical component is included. Clearly the cost would depend on the form of assessment adopted and by whom it was undertaken: whether, for example, it is seen as totally separate from existing procedures or integrated with them; undertaken by qualified social workers or social work assistants.

There are findings from the pilot study which might help to target assessment on those found not to be in need of care at the time of admission. In particular we found that those who were not in need of residential care at the time of admission were almost exclusively admitted from the community rather than from hospital. Those admitted from hospital had almost invariably already been assessed by a doctor or social worker and all that may be required by DHSS in their case is a statement that assessment has been carried out and residential care is needed. Thus, on the basis of this study, assessment could be concentrated on the 50 per cent or so of all entrants who come directly from the community, a quarter of whom might be found not in need of care. Concentrating assessment in this way might make it much more cost-effective.

Detailed work on the costs and savings of assessment remain to be undertaken in another project. However irrespective of whether it is financially worthwhile to assess everyone seeking help with residential fees through supplementary benefits there are other arguments that may well determine whether assessment of care needs is introduced:

(a)   It would introduce a greater element of public accountability.   There is widespread anxiety at present – on all sides of the political divide – that large sums of money are being spent on care that is not needed.   Assessment would allay this anxiety and reassure tax payers that public money is not being spent inappropriately.

(b)   Assessment could help to inform elderly people and their relatives about the choices available to them in making decisions about their future, and about the financial implications of different choices: between residential and community care and, when residential care is needed, between the different homes available locally in the statutory or independent sectors.

(c)   It could provide some assurance that individuals did not enter residential care unnecessarily: for want of treatment for reversible conditions or for want of support that could be supplied to them or their carers.

(d)   It could protect relatives against misjudgement of their motives or accusations that they have abandoned elderly relatives unnecessarily.

(e) Given the right administrative and financial framework it could assist local agencies to plan services for elderly people more coherently and to develop better community care 'packages'.   At the very least assessment could contribute to the development of appropriate forms of support by providing feedback on those that enable elderly people to stay at home for longer.

(f)   Assessment would increase the involvement of local authority social workers in independent homes.   This would almost certainly improve the regulation of such homes.

(g)   It could protect the private sector particularly against accusations of exploiting both the individual and the tax payer by encouraging elderly people to enter residential care unnecessarily.

There are two important counter-arguments: that making the payment of benefit in a private home dependent on the judgement of a social worker could increase the power of professionals in deciding where and how elderly people are to live, to the possible detriment of elderly people and their relatives; and that the local authority would have a gatekeeping role which gave it an unfair advantage over the independent sector inconsistent with the concept of a mixed economy of welfare.

What problems would be encountered?

The resolution of this debate will depend, in large part, on how assessment is to be operationalised. Administrative feasibility invariably plays a large part in deciding whether policies seen as desirable in principle are actually implemented. As we have stressed throughout this book a dry-run exercise such as the care needs study cannot tell us every-thing about how assessment will work in the real world. It has, nevertheless, identified many problems that would have to be resolved before it could work properly and be an improvement on the present situation. Some of these concern financial and administrative issues; some touch on professional and institutional issues; and some are more practical. The list that follows is illustrative rather than exhaustive:

(1) Assessment did work, the assessors did make judgements and it would be possible to make payment of supplementary benefit to people in homes dependent on a care assessment. However without a restructuring of financial incentives so that they are more neutral it would be unlikely to achieve all the advantages discussed earlier. As long as funding for indepen-dent residential care comes from supplementary benefit, and local authorities' funds for alternative forms of care are constrained, there will be a disincentive for local authorities to provide intensive support in the community or, arguably, to develop their own provision.

Moreover since the support required can frequently mean housing and health services as well as social and personal support it will be necessary to find ways of promoting co-operation and budget-sharing across agency boundaries locally - and Ministries centrally. (There may be much to be learned in this respect from the various experimental projects in existence around the country - notably the Kent Community Care schemes). There is now a very strong case for co-ordinating social security and community care policies.

(2) What form of assessment does DHSS want or need - and how would this relate to current practice in local authorities? The Joint Working Party recommended that assessment should be undertaken through 'existing multi-disciplinary arrangements'. In practice existing arrangements are seldom truly multi-

disciplinary and highly variable both between and within authorities. It is rarely a specialist function; there are no standard criteria; not all authorities even have assessment forms. Much of the activity presently described as assessment is actually about allocation – and may be heavily influenced by the admission criteria set by individual homes. Assessment panels, where they exist, typically consider a number of people, all judged by their individual social workers to need residential care. Because demand has until recently outstripped supply only the most urgent cases get through to the allocation process – some of whom may, ironically, be too dependent to meet the authority's or the home's admission criteria. The assessment procedures currently used for local authority accommodation do not, therefore, seem to be readily transferable to the private sector. Local authorities would have to develop a new kind of assessment capable of judging the need for residential care quite separately from decisions about entry to particular homes. For supplementary benefit purposes the type and degree of dependence would also need to be assessed in order to establish the category of care needed, and hence the level of benefit payable. Such assessments would not necessarily be once-for-all but required as often as the elderly person's conditions changed substantially. At present only the procedures used in hospitals approximate to this model.

(3) What should assessment consist of? It is likely that supplementary benefit requirements would be met by a declaration that an elderly person did or did not need residential care. However it is unthinkable that assessment, as conceived of by a professional social worker, would stop at that point. In the majority of cases further counselling or case-work would be required – either about the residential home to be chosen and the process of moving there or about alternative services. For people not already in touch with a social worker this effectively means setting up a new case file and raises questions about: who should bear the costs of such social work involvement; the extent to which elderly people want to become social work clients; the degree of social work involvement in matching clients to homes and the liabilities arising from such involvement.

(4) Would everyone entering independent care be assessed – or only those claiming SB to help meet their fees? An unknown number (17 per cent in our unrepresentative sample) of elderly people come onto supplementary benefit after they have been in homes for some time, when their capital has fallen below the £3,000 threshold. They may not need residential care, in terms of physical or mental capacity, but have no alternative to

their present placement - except a cheaper home - because they have sold their homes and lost their links with the community. If the objectives of assessment are to be fully met these people need to be assessed. However there would clearly be grave problems in requiring people not calling on public funds to be assessed prior to entering residential care. It might be possible that people with less than a given amount of capital (enough to finance them for one or perhaps two years) will be required to be assessed; or to advise all privately funded entrants to be assessed for their own peace of mind. Anything beyond this would certainly be resisted as breaching individual liberty.

(5) Crisis admissions. Admission to independent residential care is often prompted by a crisis such as the illness or death of a spouse or carer or an urgent need for a hospital bed. The time to explore the possibilities of alternatives to residential care, or set them up, is simply not available. It might be difficult to accommodate such situations in the assessment systems envisaged so far, where assessment teams might meet at intervals and waiting lists develop. Equally, however, such crises should not provide a route to independent care without full assessment. It would therefore be necessary, either to set up arrangements for short-term placement in the independent sector, while alternatives are explored; or, alternatively, for local authorities to reserve accommodation of their own for this purpose.

(6) Variability in decision-making. The assessment study found considerable variability in the proportions of elderly people judged to need residential care: between areas and between assessors working in the same area. Some of this variation will reflect real variations in the circumstances of those assessed. Need for residential care is not a cut and dried condition to be determined on the basis of some standard scale of dependency which can be applied consistently. It will depend on the elderly person's circumstances: their health and capacities; the availability of formal and informal support; their housing conditions; their own wishes and those of their carers. The judgements of assessors will reflect such factors. They will also reflect the procedures used and the criteria of need adopted by individual assessors and their authorities which we know to be highly variable between, and even within, authorities. Variation in local authority services is a familiar aspect of social policy in Britain, and defensible to the extent that it reflects differences in local populations or the preferences of the local electorate. That arising from widely differing assessment procedures is more difficult to defend and there will undoubtedly be pressure on

local authorities to standardise the methods and the criteria by which decisions are reached - not least because elderly people may wish to move to homes in other areas. What will happen, for example, when an elderly person judged by North Yorkshire to need residential care does not meet the criteria used in Devon where she wants to live? There can be no doubt that such variation will be heavily criticised, and contested, by the proprietors' associations, who are already challenging variability in registration requirements. The problem, then, is to ensure a degree of standardisation in documentation and procedures, while retaining sufficient capacity for meeting individual needs and exercising professional judgement.

(7) Will there be a right of review? The complexity of the judgements that have to be made make it more important and yet more difficult for those judgements to be opened to scrutiny. If social workers are to judge that some people who want to enter private homes do not need to and should not be funded for doing so out of public money, should the elderly people, their carers and perhaps even the homes be allowed to contest such judgements? Not to do so would represent a departure from the tradition in social security that refusal of benefit can be challenged through an independent appeal system. There is less of a tradition that social work decisions can be challenged - social workers make very important decisions at present without a right of appeal against them. However formal appeal procedures do exist in the field of child care, particuarly in the use of independent social workers as guardians ad litem. Given the anxiety among home owners in the private sector that decisions will be influenced by politically based opposition to them, and among carers that their preferences will be neglected there is a case for considering the feasibility of an independent review procedure.

The discussion of appeals is also relevant to the variability of the judgements that assessors made. While it is a methodological point within the research, it is also an important finding about the different outcomes faced by clients depending on who happens to assess them. Clearly, even with greater training and standard procedures, complete unanimity is unlikely. Greater consistency and reliability might be forthcoming if the assessments carried out by social workers were submitted to an independent body for evaluation. One such scheme operates in Canada and is discussed in greater detail in Annex 2. In the meantime, and perhaps even after the introduction of any new scheme, an appeals system will afford protection for the client and, not least, the social worker.

(8)   In the private sector the issue of assessment has aroused considerable anxiety among proprietors and their professional associations.   At a professional level, for example, some proprietors dislike the idea of a gatekeeper standing between them and their relationships with clients seeking to enter their homes.   Some do their own assessments, for example, and are unwilling to lose control of such an important task. Others are anxious about increasing the power of local authorities who are to some extent competitors.   There are fears that assessment staff employed by local authorities would direct people needing care to local authority rather than private homes;   or that those directed to private homes would be more dependent or difficult.   There is resistance to local authority staff determining the need for residential care – partly because some proprietors have experienced politically motivated hostility to the private sector among local authority staff and unions or, in some cases, from the local authority itself.   Overall then, there is some resistance to the idea of assessment by anyone other than the proprietors themselves, but particularly strong resistance to the idea that primary respon- sibility should lie with local authority social workers.   If assessment has to come, the proprietors' preference is that doctors should do it.   It could be argued that doctors are no less likely than social workers to make unbiased recommendations;   it could be argued that general practitioners have a vested interest in reducing their load of heavily depen- dent patients.   Doctors are also more expensive.   However the principal argument against using doctors is that the task of judging whether an elderly person needs residential care is one which calls primarily for social work rather than medical skills – though information on the elderly person's physical or mental capacities will be required at some stage.   Doctors are much less likely than social workers to know about the alternatives to residential care that are available in the community – to be in touch with the real prospects for community care.   This is borne out by the pilot study which found that almost a third of those found not to need residential care had been assessed by a GP before entry.   The argument about whether doctors or social workers should do assessments may, in any case, be based on a misapprehension. Assessment, if it is multi-disciplinary, will in any case involve doctors.   The anxieties of proprietors nevertheless need to be taken seriously.   Assessment could, no doubt, be imposed on the independent sector, but it would clearly be preferable to win its confidence.   It might be possible to take up the suggestion made by some proprietors that they be involved in assessment teams;   or to make the information obtained in assessment available to homes to help them to plan

care. A review procedure would be another way of allaying anxieties.

(9) If the idea of assessment is to be pursued for those wishing to enter residential care from the community consideration will need to be given to nursing homes as well. The assessors in this study stressed this point, as does Challis (1986) in a recent article. At present, with so little assessment in use, there are few controls over who receives financial help with their fees in private residential care and nursing homes. According to Challis, introducing assessment for one and not the other will merely encourage a substitution effect. Rather than remaining in the community many people will seek to enter nursing homes where the emphasis on medical care will be even less relevant to their needs. Moreover, given the fees in nursing homes, SB expenditure will rise by an amount greater than it would have done otherwise.

The next stage

The experience of the pilot study suggests that there is no intrinsic barrier to employing social workers to assess elderly people's needs for residential care in the independent sector. Social workers can make judgements about need. The decision that needs to be taken is whether, in the light of the results from the pilot study and the conclusions of the joint working party, assessment is worth pursuing. If the answer is yes, a considerable amount of thought and planning will be required before an appropriate and feasible model for assessment is developed. It will be crucial at this stage to involve, or at least consult extensively with, the interest groups involved: local authorities; social workers and their professional associations; health professionals; representatives of the private and voluntary sectors; bodies such as Age Concern and the Centre for Policy on Ageing which represent the views of elderly people and their carers. More will also need to be known at this stage about existing assessment procedures.

Once an apparently workable model has emerged there are two possible ways of proceeding. The first is to implement it immediately throughout the country and, following the conventional process of policy development in Britain, modify it in the light of experience. A more radical alternative would be to implement assessment in stages, the first stage taking the form of pilot projects in different areas. These would be evaluated and the knowledge gained used to develop the form of assessment ultimately introduced. There is not an established tradition in this country of using experiments to

assist policy development, and experiment in the field of
social security presents particular problems.   However, there
is some precedent.   Policy changes, such as the introduction
of new availability for work criteria have been preceded by
pilots.   Given the scale of the proposed changes and the
vulnerability of the client group this option certainly seems
worth considering.   To do it properly or fully might require
changes in legislation governing entitlement to SB.   However,
it would be possible to mount trials without legislative
changes if local authorities and the independent sector were to
agree to assessment of care needs being introduced.   It would
also involve the elderly being offered the choice about whether
to accept the outcome of any assessment that was carried out.

PART II
THE REASONABLENESS
OF CHARGES STUDY

7 Introduction to the charges study

Background to the research

In addition to its deliberations on assessment the Joint Working Party (DHSS 1985) was also asked:

> To consider the scope for improving collaboration between the Department of Health and Social Security (DHSS) and local authorities in relation to the support of residents in private and voluntary care homes, in particular.... ensuring that charges met from public funds are related to a reasonable standard of provision and represent value for money. (para. 1.7)

The Working Party acknowledged that DHSS local offices lacked the expertise necessary to judge what was an appropriate charge for a given standard of accommodation and care. However, they asked

> whether local authorities were not in a good position to offer advice on the level of charges which it would be reasonable for supplementary benefit to meet in particular cases. (para. 2.13)

The second main element in the research was therefore to see how personnel in social services and social work departments might set about offering advice to DHSS concerning the reasonableness of the charges being made for residential homes in the independent sector. The Joint Working Party envisaged that the local authority would draw both on their own experience in administering Part III and Part IV homes and in negotiating charges for sponsorships in the independent sector. However when we began to discuss this element of the research with local authorities in early 1986 we found them less certain than in the assessment study about whether they were equipped to undertake what they were being asked to do. This was because they were doubtful of the relevance to the independent sector of their methods of fixing charges in their own homes and, furthermore, three of the areas felt their experience of negotiating sponsorships was limited.

Charges for local authority homes were fixed as a result of an accounting exercise. The costs of all the homes in an area including capital charges were estimated and then a standard fee was fixed to meet the costs throughout all the authority's homes regardless of the facilities, services or quality of individual homes.

Of the four authorities only Lothian had any recent experience of fixing charges for sponsorship. The finance officers had fixed a charge that was considered necessary by the local authority for the home to provide a reasonable quality of service. On the basis of information provided by homeowners a figure for revenue expenditure was calculated. This included most costs related to staffing, supplies and services, administration, travel, and certain property costs such as heat and rent. A capital element was added to the figure for revenue expenditure, to take account of any requests for alterations. The latter could be built into the rate and phased over several years. Within the capital element the authority would consider, in certain cases, bank loans necessary for alterations and upgrading. However, it would not normally consider the 'capital purchase price' of the property. The figure for the revenue and capital elements, less any income from voluntary fund raising, was divided by 52 weeks and then again by a percentage based on a reasonable occupancy rate.

This process had worked well in Lothian for a number of years and most independent homes in the area had had rates set for them. However with the ending of sponsorship of new admissions the procedures had been suspended in 1985 and since then the charges for existing residents have been uprated by an index. Furthermore, the process had been lengthy, sometimes taking as long as three months from the submission of accounts. It had also been developed and maintained in a market dominated by the voluntary sector and there were grounds to doubt whether the much larger private sector outside Scotland would be willing or able to participate in the procedures. Anyway none of our other local authorities thought they had the expertise.

Devon also had experience of voluntary homes submitting their accounts with an application for an annual subvention to the local authority but this was purely an accounting exercise and did not involve setting a charge for each home based on the standard of provision. The other two authorities had limited experience of sponsorship. Sefton, for example, continued to support a small number of elderly people who were admitted before 1983 but stopped any new sponsorships after that date. So apart from Lothian the other authorities have no base of experience for assessing the reasonableness of charges.

There was also a feeling among the authorities that the amounts charged by private residential homes for the elderly were beginning to narrow – influenced by the national SB limits and the requirements of the 1984 Registered Homes Act. In the end charges were a function of demand and supply. In general, demand in the private sector tended to exceed supply. This was partly because of the availability of SB, partly because income and capital were treated more generously in the private than the public sector and partly because the standard of provision in the private sector was superior.

For these reasons it was decided to use the officers responsible for administering the provision of the Registered Homes Act 1984 and the Social Work (Scotland) Act 1968.

They do not make judgements about the reasonableness of charges at the moment. However they know most about the state of the local market – demand and supply; they inspect homes at least annually; they make several other visits; they know about and have records of the facilities offered in each home. In this sense they are better equipped than most to make judgements about the quality and range of facilities offered within a residential care home, relate it to other establishments and decide whether in comparison the charge in a particular home was reasonable.

Although this was a rather different approach to that envisaged by the Joint Working Party, with the possible exception of Lothian, we saw no practical alternative. We could have tried to tackle the issue as an accounting exercise. However, DHSS were already funding a separate costing study of private residential and nursing homes, we did not have the time or resources to mount an accounting study and we did not believe that the private homes would be willing to co-operate with one. It was therefore agreed with the steering group to the research that the reasonableness of charges study should be devoted to recording and analysing the judgements made by registration officers in each local authority.

Current legislation

In England and Wales the 1984 Registered Homes Act came fully into effect on 1 January, 1985. The new Act broadly superseded the registration provisions of two previous pieces of legislation, the Residential Homes Act, 1980, and the Nursing Homes Act, 1975. Under Part I of the new Act registration is required of any establishment providing, or intending to provide, board and personal care for persons in need of such provision. It is the responsibility of prospective proprietors to make application for registration with their local authority. The 1984 legislation also grants powers of inspection to DHSS, the Welsh Office and local authorities. The main Act is complemented by a range of other legislation. Among the most important of these are the Residential Care Homes Regulations, 1984, which deals with both the registration and conduct of such homes, and the self explanatory Registered Homes Tribunals Rules, 1984.

An integral part of the Government's measures to regulate the establishment and conduct of private and voluntary care homes was the development of a code of practice. 'Home Life: a code of practice for residential care' (Centre for Policy on Ageing 1984) sets out a philosophy of social care as well as more specific guidance on the physical features and staffing of homes and, most importantly, the rôle of registration authorities.

In Scotland the principal legislation governing registration is the Social Work (Scotland) Act, 1968. Similar to England and Wales, additional legislation in Scotland describes the form in which an application for registration is to be made, including details of the information to be provided, and sets out the procedures for hearing appeals against refusal or cancellation of registration. Although the publication of 'Home Life' has had an influence on practice outside of England and Wales, Lothian Region has published its own set of guidelines that both pre-date and anticipate much that is covered in the code of practice. Their handbook combines statements about their philosophy of care, and what is considered to be good practice, with advice on ways in which this can be achieved.

In addition to the relevant legislation and the code of practice or practice guidelines, authorities also issue notes of guidance for the registration and inspection of residential homes. Taken together, these different documents provide the framework in which homes must operate and the ground rules that determine the nature of the relationship between homes and local authorities.

The recent legislation for England and Wales has been criticised on a number of counts. Carson (1985), for example, argues that the 1984 Act pursues an accreditation model with its emphasis on minimal standards supported by sanctions of de-registration and prosecution. Of particular relevance to reasonableness of charges, Carson suggests that an alternative approach could have included 'procedures akin to rent regulation so that charges could be assessed against the accommodation and services provided'. Others have also commented on the lack of provision in the Act for local authorities to see all the financial documents of a private residential home applying for registration (Bingley, 1986). The Act is also seen as ineffective in dealing with homes that fail to register. An authority may prosecute such a home but it cannot, under present legislation, close it down.

8 Registration and residential care homes

The role of registration officers

We have referred to the people involved in this study throughout the report as registration officers although their duties, in addition to registration, frequently involve inspection. Where they perform both tasks, as they do in three authorities in this study, the term 'registration and inspection officer' is probably more precise. However, in some authorities, officers specialize in one rôle or the other. Sefton, for example, have appointed two registration officers and two inspection officers who work as a team in spite of the division of labour.

The relevant legislation in Britain has laid general responsibility on local authorities to ensure that standards of care in residential homes meet at least prescribed minimal requirements. They also have a duty to ensure that residents are offered the best quality of life. Registration officers are responsible therefore for making sure that these obligations are properly discharged.

There are three main areas of registration. The first relates to prospective homes that seek to open in an area; the second to existing homes that wish to register for additional categories of care; and the third to those homes where a change of ownership is intended. The first is probably the most time consuming of the three, involving considerable consultation with other related agencies such as the district planning authority, environmental health and fire service. However, even before these checks are carried out, registration officers provide the first point of contact between the prospective home owner and the registering authority. During this pre-registration period many authorities send out packs which set out in detail the requirements for registration. Some registration officers will provide advice, among other things, on the general financial implications of establishing a new home. This is especially important where substantial loans are necessary to start a home. In Southport, for example, the average borrowing of new proprietors in 1986 was between £120,000 and £150,000 which, in turn, required an average monthly repayment to the bank of £1800 (Murray, 1986). Registration officers are not in a position to offer specialist financial advice, home owners must seek this from accountants, but they can say whether the proposed charge is reasonable in the light of the local market conditions.

Once an authority has granted registration (and it is the authority not the registration officer who is responsible for this) registration officers will then undertake inspection, monitoring and support. It is not uncommon for a new home to be visited within three months of being established. Thereafter homes will be visited at least once a year for a formal comprehensive review which will identify any issues or items that need attention. Registration officers involved with this project have stressed the importance of improving standards by consultation and advice rather than rigid dictat. This consultative and gradualist approach is part of the partnership that many authorities are attempting to establish with homes (Shipley, 1985).

Broadly speaking therefore, registration officers are engaged in the following activities:

(a) Providing preliminary advice to prospective proprietors.

(b) Inspecting premises prior to registration.

(c) Liaising with other statutory agencies to ensure standards and compliance with other legislation.

(d) Co-ordinating the procedures necessary for the local authority to approve registration.

(e) Inspecting homes on a regular basis after registration.

(f) Providing support and advice.

Brooke Ross (1985) provides a detailed discussion of the regulation of residential homes in general, and Fryer (1985) examines the registration process operating in Leicestershire.

The Registration Officers

In this study the assessment of reasonableness of charges was carried out by ten registration officers, covering between 15 and 31 homes each. There were four officers working on assessments in Sefton, three in Devon, two in Lothian and one in Clwyd. The six men and four women came to their present posts from a variety of social work and residential care backgrounds. Three were graduates, eight were qualified social workers holding the CQSW or its equivalent, and four had qualifications in residential social work or residential care. Six of the group had fieldwork experience, eight had experience in residenital settings and five, at some stage, had held management posts connected with residential care.

It was intended that the registration officers would complete a questionnaire for each home visited as part of the assessment of care needs study. In principle we should have received 182 questionnaires, in reality 222 were completed, mainly due to a misunderstanding in one area. Table 8.1 provides a summary of the number of questionnaires completed by each registration officer.

Table 8.1
Number of questionnaires completed by each registration officer

		%	N		%	N
Lothian	1	8.1	18	)		
	2	8.1	18	)	16.2	36
Devon	1	14.0	31	)		
	2	6.7	15	)	32.9	73
	3	12.2	27	)		
Sefton	1	9.0	20	)		
	2	9.9	22	)		
	3	7.6	17	)	38.7	86
	4	12.2	27	)		
Clwyd	1	12.2	27		12.2	27
Totals		100.0	222		100.0	222

The registration officers attended a briefing in York at the beginning of October 1986. The focus of the meeting was the latest version of a questionnaire to be completed by them for specified homes in their area. A number of amendments arising from the discussion were incorporated into the final version of the reasonableness of charges questionnaire. Registration officers received this at the end of October, and started work almost straight away. No written instructions or guidance for completing the questionnaire was issued as registration officers felt that the task, while time-consuming, was reasonably straightforward.

Before starting work on the exercise registration officers, using a draft letter prepared by the research team, wrote to every owner and manager in their area likely to feature in the reasonableness of charges study. The letter, additional to the one sent by DHSS at the start of the study, thanked home owners and managers for their help in the assessment study and informed them of the nature and purpose of the reasonableness of charges study. The letter also indicated that the research was not concerned with the identity of individual homes.

The sample of homes

In Table 8.2 we find that overall the homes assessed represented 122 per cent of those containing people included in the assessment study and 86 per cent of all homes in the area. These proportions varied, with the coverage in Sefton being considerably higher than the coverage in Lothian.

Of the residential care homes included in the study 19.8 per cent were voluntary. However, this again varied from area to area. In Lothian, as Table 8.3 indicates, two thirds of the homes assessed were voluntary.

Table 8.2
Homes in the reasonableness of charges study

	1 No. of ind. homes in in area in area N	2 No. with clients in the assess-ment study N	% of 1	3 No. in charges study N	% of 2	% of 1
Lothian	50	37	74.0	36[1]	97.3	72.0
Devon	83	70	84.3	73[2]	104.3	88.0
Sefton	89	48	53.9	86[3]	179.2	96.6
Clwyd	36	27	75.0	27	100.0	75.0
Totals	258	182	70.5	222	122.0	86.0

Notes:

1 Registration officers in Lothian did not complete a questionnaire for one home, which was in the process of closing

2 Registration officers in Devon completed three extra questionnaires for homes that had not featured in the assessment of care needs study

3 Registration officers in Sefton completed a questionnaire for nearly every home in Southport even though many of the homes had not featured in the assessment of care needs study

Table 8.3
Type of home by area

	Lothian N	Devon N	Sefton N	Clwyd N	All N	%
Private home	11	68	74	25	178	80.2
Voluntary home	25	5	12	2	44	19.8
Totals	36	73	86	27	222	

Registration officers relied to a considerable extent on their records in carrying out the assessments. These were mainly derived from the statutory annual inspection carried out under the 1984 Registered Homes Act and the 1968 Social Work (Scotland) Act. We had expected that all homes would have been inspected within one year of the start of the study. From Table 8.4 fourteen of the homes appeared not to have been inspected for over a year. Further enquiries revealed that most in fact had been inspected within the last year but there had been a delay in bringing the relevant records up-to-date. There is also an important distinction between unannounced visits, and full inspections. In most cases, homes would have been visited at least once, probably twice, in the previous year, and the records updated as appropriate. Because the registration records for a small minority of homes were not up-to-date the registration officers did not rely entirely on them - nine homes were visited especially for the study and telephone calls were made to supplement the records in six cases.

Table 8.4
Time since last registration inspection

	N	%
After September 1986	2	(2)
September 1986	25	11.3
August 1986	38	17.1
February–July 1986	73	32.9
September 1985–January 1986	70	31.5
Over a year previously	14	6.3
Totals	222	100.0

The reasonableness of charges questionnaire

It was originally envisaged that the questionnaire would be completed by registration officers on the basis of a special visit to the home. Registration officers dismissed this proposal as unrealistic. Given the time and resources available they were only willing to complete the questionnaire from information contained in the last annual inspection report. This had implications of course for the design and coverage of the questionnaire. In essence the questionnaire was limited to previously recorded information. The judgements that registration officers would be asked to make would likewise be limited to this information. In practice the annual inspection documents in use in each authority were comprehensive in their coverage and we were able to obtain most of the information that was required from them.

The questionnaire contained three sections and 35 questions, considerably shorter than the instrument used in the assessment study. The first section was concerned with background information about the home. In particular, private or voluntary; when first registered; whether any part was purpose built; type of resident; size; charges for different sized rooms; and details of a range of other facilities. The second section asked registration officers to rate and comment on various features of the home, including local area, gardens, decorative order, quality of care, atmosphere and catering. They were also asked about the staff and asked to provide an overall rating of the home. The final section focused on the reasonableness of the charges and the criteria employed in making a judgement of this kind. Registration officers were also asked to indicate the main sources of their information and the amount of time required for each.

As with the assessment study, the questionnaire was discussed within the research unit and also externally with registration officers and DHSS. Again, there was no opportunity to pilot the questionnaire.

9 Residential care homes and charges

Characteristics of the homes

Most of the 222 homes in the sample had been running for a comparatively short time; 189 had started operating since 1970 and 106 of these since 1980. Only three of the homes were operating before the last war. While only seven homes were purpose built for residential care of the elderly a further 38 had purpose built extensions. Prior to operating as residential homes two-thirds (142) of the buildings had been private houses or flats and 42 (19 per cent) had been hotels or guest houses.

Table 9.1 provides a breakdown of the number of residents homes in each area were permitted to take at the time of the survey. Just over 20 per cent were registered to take ten or fewer residents — two homes were registered for four beds, the threshold at which registration is required. Devon had significantly more smaller homes than Lothian and Clwyd. About half the homes were permitted to take between 11 and 20 residents and a further 20 per cent were registered for 21-30 residents. Overall, less than 12 per cent of homes were permitted to take more than 30 residents. However, many of the larger homes were to be found in Lothian; Devon and Sefton in particular had their smallest proportion of homes in this category.

Table 9.1
Number of residents permitted in homes

Area	Size 4-10		11-20		21-30		Over 30		Totals	
	N	%	N	%	N	%	N	%	N	Mean
Lothian	4	11.4	14	40.0	6	17.1	11	31.5	35	27.3
Devon	21	28.8	30	41.1	19	26.0	3	4.1	73	16.4
Sefton	18	20.9	45	52.3	15	17.5	8	9.3	86	17.8
Clwyd	4	14.8	15	55.6	4	14.8	4	14.8	27	21.3
Totals	47	21.3	104	47.1	44	19.9	26	11.8	221	19.3

Missing cases= 1

At their last inspection over half (58 per cent) of the homes had vacancies, with 23 having more than five and one of these as many as 18. At the other extreme 92 (42 per cent) homes were fully occupied.

From this data we calculated two occupancy rates. The first was the number in residence at the last annual inspection as a proportion of the number of residents plus vacancies - the true rate. The second was the number in residence at the last inspection as a proportion of the number the home was permitted to take - the theoretical rate.

There was little difference between the occupancy rates using either measure. The true rate was 89 per cent and the theoretical rate 86 per cent. Table 9.2 shows that occupancy varied from 95 per cent in Lothian to 86 per cent in Devon. The difference between the true and theoretical rates was also largest in Devon suggesting that the market in Devon is more competitive than in other areas. Voluntary homes had higher occupancy rates than private homes. Those whose charges were considered unreasonable had slightly lower occupancy rates and also homes whose overall assessment was only adequate or poor had lower occupancy rates than the others.

Table 9.2
Occupancy rates

	Mean %	SD	N
True occupancy rate	88.61	(15.2)	220
Theoretical occupancy rate	86.10	(16.0)	222

True occupancy rates

	Mean %	SD	N
Lothian	95.36	(7.4)	36
Devon	86.21	(17.5)	72
Sefton	88.03	(15.7)	85
Clwyd	87.88	(12.8)	27

	Mean %	SD	N
Private homes	87.86	(16.0)	176
Voluntary homes	92.32	(10.0)	44

	Mean %	SD	N
Charges reasonable	80.88	(15.6)	179
Charges too high	86.72	(14.6)	34
Charges too low	90.95	(8.9)	7

Overall assessment of home

	Mean %	SD	N
Poor	87.78	(14.0)	11
Adequate	85.48	(16.5)	50
Good	89.09	(15.6)	82
Very good	90.56	(14.7)	66
Excellent	90.46	(11.1)	11

Missing cases= 2

Charges and differential charging

Charges vary - they vary between homes and within homes for the same type of room and for different rooms. As our data covers a period of over a year, charges also vary over time. They can also vary in homes registered to take different categories with the degree of dependency of the resident. In addition as we shall see, homes may charge more or less for SB residents. Making sense of, and summarising, all this variation is not easy.

In Table 9.3 we start by presenting data on the minimum and maximum being charged in the homes. The lowest minimum was £45 being charged by a voluntary home in Devon for a single room. The highest minimum was £175 per week being charged by a private home in Sefton. The lowest maximum was again £45 for the same voluntary home in Devon and the highest maximum was £300 being charged for a bed in a double room by a private home in Devon (this figure was confirmed by the registration officer). The mean minimum charge was £117 and the mean maximum was £133.

Table 9.3
Range of charges

	Lowest	Highest	Mean	(SD)
Minimum	£45	£175	£116.77	(18.7)
Maximum	£45	£300	£133.33	(28.8)

Table 9.4 provides details of charging structures for the homes. A third of the homes had varying charges for the same type of room. In just less than a third the homes charged the same regardless of the type of room. There was some variation in charging structure between areas with Devon and Clwyd having rather variable charges and Lothian having more stable ones.

Table 9.5 shows how the mean minimum and maximum charges varied between areas and private and voluntary homes. On average voluntary homes had both lower minima and maxima.

However, it is interesting to note that the mean minimum in Lothian, which has a higher proportion of voluntary homes, is higher than the other areas. This is because the few private homes in Lothian tended to have relatively high minimum charges and, furthermore, charges which tended not to vary by type of room. While the minimum and maximum charge in Lothian was almost identical, the other areas had greater variation with the mean minimum and maximum in Devon varying by £31.

Table 9.4
Charging structure

	Lothian % N=36	Devon % N=73	Sefton % N=86	Clwyd % N=27	All (%) N=222
Homes where min. and max. are the same for the same type of room	38.9	6.8	20.9	–	37 (16.7)
Homes where min. and max. are the same for different types of room	52.8	9.6	40.7	14.8	65 (29.3)
Homes where min. and max. are different for different types of room	2.8	43.8	11.6	11.1	46 (20.7)
Homes where min. and max. are different for same type of room	5.5	39.7	26.7	74.1	74 (33.3)
Totals	100.0	100.0	100.0	100.0	100.0

x^2= 95.38   P<0.0001

Table 9.5
Range of charges by area and type of home

	Minimum (£ mean)	(SD)	Maximum (£ mean)	(SD)	N
Lothian	126	(18.3)	127	(17.8)	36
Devon	114	(18.1)	145	(36.1)	73
Sefton	117	(20.6)	126	(26.2)	86
Clwyd	113	(8.0) p<0.001	131	(12.8) p<0.001	27
Private	119.46	(15.7)	139.08	(25.7)	178
Voluntary	105.89	(25.2) p<0.001	108.36	(27.7) p<0.001	44
All	117	(18.7)	133	(28.8)	222

Table 9.6 gives a frequency distribution of the minimum and maximum charges for the homes in the study. It is notable that the minimum charge in 39 per cent of homes was £120 or £125, the SB limit during the assessment period for homes registered to care for the elderly. By controlling for the date of the last registration inspection, we find that the minimum charge in 73.9 per cent of homes was at, or below, the SB limit for the elderly. Of those with minimum charges over the elderly limit we found no homes registered for non elderly categories. Therefore 36 per cent of homes had a minimum charge which was more than the SB limit for their category of home.

Table 9.6
Minimum and maximum charges

Minimum charges (£)	%	N
Up to 100	17.1	38
101–119	22.5	50
120	22.1	49
121–124	1.8	4
125	17.1	38
126–129	1.8	4
130+	17.6	39
Totals	100.0	222

Maximum charges (£)	%	N
Up to 100	8.6	19
101–119	10.4	23
120	14.2	31
121–124	1.8	4
125	9.9	22
126–129	1.4	3
130	7.7	17
131–139	7.2	16
140	13.1	29
141–149	3.6	8
150	7.2	16
150+	15.3	34
Totals	100.0	222

There was one home which admitted to charging more for new residents in receipt of SB compared with the charge for other residents. It was a voluntary home in Lothian charging SB cases £125 and private residents £101 on the grounds that the DHSS maximum justified the higher charge. There were 18 homes charging less for new residents on SB and 20 homes charging less for existing residents. (See Table 9.7) In four cases the owners justified charging less on the basis of room size, facilities and views, ie., they indicated that SB recipients were being charged less because they occupied inferior accommodation. However in the other cases the differential charge was justified on the grounds that DHSS would not pay more than the limit (four cases), the needs of the person (1 case) and non SB residents being charged as much as the market can bear (1 case).

Table 9.7
Differential charging

	New residents		Long stay residents	
	N	%	N	%
Those on SB charged more	1	0.5	–	0.0
Those on SB charged less	18	8.3	20	9.3
Those on SB charged the same	195	89.8	190	89.2
No-one on SB	3	1.4	3	1.4
Totals	217	100.0	213	100.0
Missing cases=	5		9	

So far we have looked at the minimum and maximum charges for the homes. We now turn to examine the charges made for rooms within the homes. The type of accommodation available within the homes and the charges for the rooms is summarised in Table 9.8. Of the homes 95 per cent had single rooms with charges varying from £45 to £250 per week (min. mean= £120 per week). About 41 per cent of these homes had differential charges for their single rooms. Eighty-four per cent of the homes contained double rooms with charges varying from £77 to £300 per week. About 29 per cent of these homes had differential charges for double rooms. A much smaller proportion of homes had multi-bedded rooms - 17 per cent with three bedded rooms and seven per cent with rooms with more than three beds. These tended to be voluntary homes in Lothian but there was one private home in Sefton charging £175 per bed in rooms with more than three beds. (This home had 34 bed spaces all charged at £175 per week - 29 were occupied providing an annual income of £264,000 per annum. The registration officer considered that the fees were excessive).

Table 9.8
Charges for rooms

	Min. £	Max. £	% with a differential charge	Min. Mean £	Max. Mean £	N	%
Single rooms	45	250	41.4	120.11	131.05	210	94.6
Double rooms	77	300	29.0	119.57	126.81	186	83.8
Rooms with 3 beds	65	165	15.8	120.32	124.40	38	17.1
Rooms with more than 3 beds	65	175	(1)	122.81	125.63	16	7.2
All	45	300				222	

10 Assessment of reasonableness of charges

The rating of the home

The questionnaire used for assessing the reasonableness of charges asked for information on a number of features of the residential home. The registration officers were asked to reflect on this information, their knowledge of the homes and their own records and rate the homes on the following factors:

Factors	Weighting/Relative importance
(1) Local area	Low
(2) Upkeep of garden and exterior of property	Low
(3) Decorative order and standard of furnishing	Low
(4) Range and quality of facilities	Medium
(5) Presence of experienced staff	Medium
(6) Quality of care	High
(7) Atmosphere within the home	Medium
(8) Catering	Low
(9) Turnover of staff	Low
(10) Competence of staff	Medium
(11) Amount of on-going training	Medium

From the rating of the 11 factors above, and further information provided by registration officers about the relative importance they placed on each, raw and weighted overall rating scores were generated. Alpha coefficients were calculated for the two scales as measures of their reliability or internal consistency. Coefficients in excess of 0.87 were found for both the raw and weighted scales, an indication that sufficient internal consistency existed for the sum of the individual items to be taken as a reliable measure.

Registration officers were then asked 'taking into account all the things that you would consider important, how would you assess this home' - poor, adequate, good, very good, excellent. This variable is referred to as the 'overall assessment' to distinguish it from the raw and weighted rating scores.

The results derived from the raw and weighted rating scores and the overall assessment are given in Table 10.1. Five per cent of homes were assessed as poor and five per cent as excellent. The majority of homes were good or better but just over a quarter were only adequate or poor. [With the agreement of the registration officers, a classification of adequate represented "just about meeting the minimal requirements for registration"]. Both raw and weighted rating scores increased directly in line with the overall assessment.

Table 10.1
Overall assessment by rating scores

Overall assessment	N	%	Rating scales			
			Raw score		Weighted score	
			Mean	S.D.	Mean	S.D.
Poor	11	5.0	15.4	(1.7)	30.7	(4.2)
Adequate	51	23.0	20.7	(2.5)	42.4	(5.0)
Good	83	37.4	24.4	(2.3)	51.2	(4.8)
Very good	66	29.6	29.4	(2.5)	61.1	(4.2)
Excellent	11	5.0	33.4	(1.5)	69.4	(3.5)
All	222	100.0	25.1	(4.9)	52.0	(10.1)

$p < 0.001$ $p < 0.001$

At first sight there is a paradox that 11 homes judged suitable for registration should be seen in this exercise as 'poor' and not meeting adequate standards. Further enquiries revealed that authorities were either in the process of cancelling the registration of 'poor' homes, or the homes in question had been set a deadline for meeting minimum standards.

Table 10.2
Variation in the rating of the homes

		% rated adequate or poor	% rated v. good or excellent	Raw rating score (Mean)	(SD)	Weighted rating score (Mean)	(SD)	N
Registration officer								
Lothian	1	16.7	66.7	28.5	(5.3)	57.4	(10.1)	18
	2	22.2	55.5	27.7	(5.3)	56.3	(11.4)	18
Devon	1	25.8	25.8	23.6	(3.6)	48.4	(6.8)	31
	2	40.0	20.0	22.7	(2.6)	48.3	(6.8)	15
	3	22.2	48.1	28.0	(4.5)	56.1	(10.5)	27
Sefton	1	30.0	30.0	24.7	(4.9)	51.1	(9.9)	20
	2	4.5	54.5	26.7	(3.4)	57.1	(6.7)	22
	3	64.7	11.8	22.6	(5.8)	46.1	(11.6)	17
	4	18.5	22.2	25.5	(4.2)	53.2	(8.5)	27
Clywd	1	44.4	18.5	22.6	(4.9)	47.0	(11.0)	27
		p<0.001		p<0.001		p<0.001		
Area								
Lothian		19.4	61.1	28.1	(5.2)	56.9	(10.6)	36
Devon		27.4	32.8	25.0	(4.4)	51.1	(9.1)	73
Sefton		26.7	30.2	25.1	(4.7)	52.4	(4.6)	86
Clwyd		44.4	18.5	22.6	(4.9)	47.0	(11.0)	27
		p<0.01		p<0.001		p<0.001		
Type of home								
Private		29.2	29.7	24.7	(4.8)	51.1	(10.2)	178
Voluntary		20.5	54.6	27.5	(4.6)	56.1	(8.7)	44
		p<0.05		p<0.001		p<0.001		
All		28.0	34.7	25.2	(4.9)	52.0	(10.1)	222

Table 10.2 shows how the assessment of the homes varied by registration officer, area and type of home. Homes in Clwyd were assessed least well on average but the least generous assessments were given by one of the registration officers in Sefton who considered that 65 per cent of the homes in his area were only adequate or poor. The most favourably assessed homes were in Lothian where one of the registration officers thought that over two thirds of the homes were very good or excellent. On average voluntary homes received more favourable assessments than private homes.

The obvious question to ask about these results is do the variations reflect real differences between the homes or differences in the judgements of the registration officers? An inspection of the scores and overall assessment given by the different registration officers indicates the assessments are in fact quite consistent.

Table 10.3 examines the relationship between charges and the overall assessment of the care home in two ways. First the mean charge is broken down by the overall assessment ranging from 'poor' to 'excellent'. The mean charge for poor and adequate homes tends to be lower than that for good and excellent homes but the differences are very slight. Secondly, the correlations between the charges and the raw and weighted rating scores, reveal no discernible relationships.

In case this might be because we had four different local residential care home markets and two types of home, we carried out the analysis for private homes only for each area. The results in Table 10.4 show that excluding voluntary homes tends to alter the direction of the correlation but does not improve its strength. The only correlations which were statistically significant at the one per cent level are between the raw ratings and the minimum and maximum charges for private homes considered to be charging reasonable amounts. But even then the coefficients were no more than r= 0.221. This preliminary analysis suggests therefore that there is very little relationship between registration officers' rating of the home and the charges made by the home.

Table 10.3
Overall assessment and charges

Overall assess- ment	Minimum charge			Minimum charge for a single room			Minimum charge for a double room			Maximum charge		
	Mean £	(SD)	N	Mean £	(SD)	N	Mean £	(SD)	N	Mean £	(SD)	N
Poor	115	(26)	11	117	(25)	11	122	(22)	9	127	(35)	11
Adequate	117	(17)	51	122	(17)	50	122	(20)	46	135	(21)	51
Good	116	(17)	83	120	(20)	77	117	(15)	70	131	(24)	83
Very good	117	(21)	66	119	(22)	62	120	(22)	52	132	(37)	66
Excellent	125	(13)	11	125	(14)	10	124	(14)	9	146	(27)	11
All	117	(19)	222	120	(20)	210	120	(18)	186	133	(29)	222
	NS			NS			NS			NS		
Correlation with raw rating score	0.024 p=0.361			−0.034 p=0.311			−0.029 p=0.345			0.033 p=0.314		
Correlation with weighted rating score	0.006 p=0.464			−0.050 p=0.238			−0.051 p=0.248			−0.012 p=0.431		

Table 10.4
Correlation between charges and ratings - private homes

	Raw rating scores		Weighted rating scores		
	R	p	R	p	N
Lothian					
Min. charge for single	-0.025	0.471	-0.044	0.450	11
Min. charge for double	-0.225	0.253	-0.220	0.258	11
Devon					
Min. charge for single	0.103	0.201	0.132	0.144	68
Min. charge for double	-0.035	0.389	-0.070	0.286	68
Sefton					
Min. charge for single	-0.069	0.280	-0.105	0.189	74
Min. charge for double	-0.055	0.321	0.024	0.419	74
Clwyd					
Min. charge for single	-0.070	0.370	-0.092	0.332	25
Min. charge for double	-0.120	0.285	-0.197	0.173	25
Min. charge - ALL	0.101	0.090	0.088	0.123	178
Max. charge - ALL	0.163	0.015	0.107	0.079	178
Min. charge for single	-0.045	0.274	-0.061	0.212	178
Min. charge for double	-0.096	0.100	-0.077	0.154	178
Charge considered reasonable					
Min. charge - ALL	0.195	0.010	0.188	0.013	143
Max. charge - ALL	0.221	0.004	0.153	0.035	143

The facilities in the home

The questionnaire also asked about the different facilities available within homes. Whereas registration officers made a judgement about the factors outlined above, they were only asked to say whether a facility, such as chiropody, was available within the home, or how many people shared a particular facility. At this stage no form of rating or assessment was involved. From the following list of items it was possible to construct a raw or unweighted index of facilities:

	Facilities	Weighting/ relative importance
(1)	Single rooms	High
(2)	Baths	Medium
(3)	WCs	High
(4)	Sitting rooms	High
(5)	Call system	High
(6)	Lift	Medium
(7)	Hairdressing	Low
(8)	Chiropody	Low
(9)	Physiotherapy	Low
(10)	Occupational therapy	Low

At a later stage registration officers were asked about the relative importance they placed on each facility. On the basis of this information it was then possible to construct a weighted index of facilities.

The raw and weighted indices yielded alpha coefficients of less than 0.40, an indication that there existed little internal consistency between the individual items. However, given that we were not attempting to measure attitudes, where internal consistency between items is essential before employing a global score, the relatively low alpha coefficients did not prevent us from using the raw and weighted indices of facilities in our analysis.

As a starting point we examined the relationship between facilities and the overall rating and assessment measures outlined in the previous section. Table 10.5 shows quite clearly that there is a modest but statistically positive relationship between the registration officers' assessment of the homes and the facilities within it.

Table 10.5
Correlation between ratings, overall assessment and facilities

Indices of facilities

	Raw scores		Weighted scores		
	R	p	R	p	N
Raw rating score	0.338	0.001	0.316	0.001	222
Weighted rating score	0.333	0.001	0.318	0.001	222
Overall assessment	0.330	0.001	0.334	0.001	222

We then examined more closely the relationship between the facilities and the overall assessment. The results set out in Table 10.6 indicate that both raw and weighted indices of facilities increased directly in line with registration officers' overall assessment of homes.

Table 10.6
Overall assessment by facilities

Overall assessment	N	%	Indices of facilities			
			Raw score		Weighted score	
			Mean	SD	Mean	SD
Poor	11	5.0	5.8	1.6	13.3	5.6
Adequate	51	23.0	5.9	1.3	13.3	4.0
Good	83	37.4	6.5	1.2	16.0	3.7
Very good	66	29.6	7.0	1.5	16.8	4.2
Excellent	11	5.0	7.4	1.1	18.1	3.0
All	222		6.5	1.4	15.6	4.3
			$p < 0.001$		$p < 0.001$	

Table 10.7 sets out the results for the variation in the raw and weighted indices of facilities. There was no significant difference between the four authorities for the two indices of facilities. The overall mean scores for private and voluntary homes were also very similar.

Table 10.8 examines whether the charges in a home are related to its facilities. On the basis of all homes in the sample the relationship is weak and barely discernible. Again, in case this might have been a reflection of four different local residential care homes markets, and two types of homes in the independent sector, we limited the analyses to private homes for each area. Although the correlation coefficients increase slightly none are statistically significant at the one per cent level. In the light of this evidence it is not unreasonable to conclude that there exists no necessary relationship between the facilities within a home and the charges made by the home.

Table 10.7
Facilities by area and type of home

Indices of facilities

Type of home	Raw score Mean	(SD)	Weighted score Mean	(SD)	N
Area					
Lothian	6.7	(1.5)	16.2	(4.3)	36
Devon	6.6	(1.3)	15.8	(3.8)	73
Sefton	6.3	(1.5)	14.9	(4.6)	86
Clwyd	6.8	(1.2)	16.1	(4.2)	27
	NS		NS		
Type of home					
Private	6.4	(1.4)	15.4	(4.3)	178
Voluntary	6.9	(1.4)	16.2	(4.1)	44
	NS		NS		
All	6.5	(1.4)	15.6	(4.3)	222

Before considering the reasonableness of charges it is worth summarising the main findings so far. Whereas the rating and overall assessment of a home, and the facilities within a home, were related to one another, these measures were found to have very little relationship with charges.

Reasonableness of charges

The judgement that the registration officers made about the reasonableness of charges in the home was a general one. That is it was not made in relation to a particular individual with a given level of dependency. Nor was it made in respect of the minimum or maximum charge where this varied. It was a general judgement of the average charge in the home.

The registration officers thought that the basic charge was reasonable in 82 per cent of the homes. In seven homes (3.2 per cent) they considered too little was being charged and in 34 homes (15.3 per cent) too much was being charged.

Table 10.8
Correlation between charges and facilities

Indices of facilities

ALL HOMES (Private and Voluntary)	Raw scores R	p	Weighted score R	p	N
Min. charge - ALL	-0.094	0.081	-0.093	0.083	222
Max. charge - ALL	0.006	0.465	-0.028	0.340	222
Min. charge for single room	0.082	0.112	0.035	0.304	222
Min. charge for double room	-0.022	0.374	-0.076	0.129	222

PRIVATE HOMES ONLY

Lothian					
Min. charge for single	0.245	0.234	0.341	0.153	11
Min. charge for double	-0.247	0.232	-0.239	0.240	11
Devon					
Min. charge for single	-0.114	0.177	-0.210	0.043	68
Min. charge for double	0.474	0.351	0.078	0.263	68
Sefton					
Min. charge for single	0.145	0.109	0.046	0.350	74
Min. charge for double	0.043	0.360	-0.103	0.190	74
Clwyd					
Min. charge for single	-0.075	0.361	-0.036	0.433	25
Min. charge for double	-0.079	0.354	-0.156	0.229	25
Min. charge - ALL	-0.134	0.037	-0.156	0.020	178
Max. charge - ALL	0.050	0.254	-0.028	0.354	178
Min. charge for single room	0.097	0.099	0.029	0.349	178
Min. charge for double room	0.041	0.293	-0.031	0.343	178

Charges considered reasonable

	Raw scores R	p	Weighted score R	p	N
Min. charge - ALL	-0.046	0.294	-0.057	0.250	143
Max. charge - ALL	0.099	0.121	0.019	0.413	143

The results are presented in Table 10.9. There was some variation in the proportions judged as unreasonable by different registration officers. Thus for example Sefton 3 thought 29 per cent of the homes he visited were charging too much – while his colleague Sefton 2 considered that only 14 per cent were charging too much. Most striking is the one registration officer in Clwyd who considered 37 per cent of his homes were charging too much and 15 per cent were charging too little. The proportion charging too much was not significantly different in Lothian and Devon – about eight per cent. Private homes were more likely than voluntary homes to be charging too much but voluntary homes were more likely to be charging too little.

Table 10.9
Reasonableness of charges

	Reasonable %	Too much %	Too little %	N	
Lothian 1	100.0	–	–	18	
2	83.3	16.7	–	18	
Devon 1	83.9	9.7	6.5	31	
2	93.3	6.7	–	15	
3	88.9	7.4	3.7	27	
Sefton 1	85.0	15.0	–	20	
2	86.4	13.6	–	22	
3	70.6	29.4	–	17	
4	85.2	14.8	–	27	
Clywd	48.1	37.0	14.8	27	p<0.01
Lothian	91.7	8.3	–	36	
Devon	87.7	8.2	4.1	73	
Sefton	82.6	17.4	–	86	
Clwyd	48.1	37.0	14.8	27	p<0.001
Private	80.3	18.0	1.7	178	
Voluntary	86.4	4.5	9.1	44	p<0.01
Totals	81.5	15.3	3.2	100.0	
N	181	34	7	222	

In Table 9.10 we compare the mean charges of the homes. As one might expect, the lowest mean charges are for those homes that the registration officer considered too low and the highest charges for those they considered too high. However there is some overlap between charges considered reasonable and those considered too high.

Table 10.10
Charges

	Min. charge £	(SD)	N
Reasonable	116.27	(18.2)	181
Too much	124.18	(15.9)	34
Too little	93.71	(24.9)	7
All	116.77	(18.7)	222 (p<0.001)

	Max. charge £	(SD)	N
Reasonable	131.91	(28.1)	181
Too much	145.35	(25.1)	34
Too little	100.86	(35.4)	7
All	132.99	(28.8)	222 (p<0.001)

Minimum for a single room	£	(SD)	N
Reasonable	119.53	(18.4)	169
Too much	128.41	(20.0)	34
Too little	93.71	(24.9)	7
All	120.10	(19.7)	210 (p<0.001)

Minimum for a double room	£	(SD)	N
Reasonable	118.66	(18.1)	148
Too much	127.09	(19.1)	32
Too little	101.83	(13.9)	6
All	119.56	(18.7)	186 (p<0.01)

Homes with reasonable charges

Three of these homes had minimum charges in excess of £150 per week and 34 (19.1 per cent) of the sample had charges in excess of £125, the current DHSS limit for the elderly. The highest charge considered reasonable was £170 per week.

If DHSS were to pay charges that registration officers considered reasonable then the minimum charges being paid for SB recipients in 15.3 per cent of the homes would have increased by an average of £13.68.

Homes charging too much

Table 10.11 shows, for those homes charging too much, the excess of their charge over what the registration officer thought was reasonable. One home had a minimum charge £45 above what was considered reasonable. However the minimum charge considered reasonable was on average only £14.07 lower than the minimum charge and only £36.73 below the maximum charge.

Table 10.11
Excess of charge over reasonable charge:
homes charging too much

Minimum charge too much		Maximum charge too much	
£	N	£	N
-10	1	10	2
-5	1	14	1
0	5	17	1
5	4	20	5
10	4	25	5
15	2	30	5
17	1	35	2
20	4	37	1
25	4	40	2
30	1	45	1
35	1	50	2
40	1	54	1
45	1	60	1
		70	2
		75	1
		100	1

Mean excess: £14.07 (13.5) 30   £36.73 (21.8) 30

Table 10.12 compares the difference between the charges considered unreasonable and the DHSS limit (in this case the pre-July limit for the elderly of £120 per week is taken). One home had a minimum charge £55 over the limit and two homes with maximum charges £80 above the limit. However there were nine homes whose charges were considered unreasonable, whose minimum charge was less than the limit, and eight homes were on the limit. On average the minimum charge exceeded the limit by only £4.18.

Table 10.12
Excess of charge over £120: homes charging too much

Minimum charge		Maximum charge	
£	N	£	N
-20	2	-20	1
-15	1	-5	1
-10	6	0	5
0	8	5	3
5	8	14	1
10	3	17	1
20	2	20	9
22	1	22	1
30	1	30	2
40	1	40	3
55	1	55	3
		59	1
		75	1
		80	2
Mean	4.18	Mean	25.35
(SD)	(15.9)	(SD)	(25.1)
N=34		N=34	

If the DHSS were to pay only charges that the registration office thought reasonable then the 15 per cent of homes charging too much could expect reductions of £14.07 per week on average for their minimum charges. However a few homes would still be charging over the present limits. Table 10.13 shows the charges that registration officers thought were reasonable for homes charging too much - in two cases reasonable charges were considered to be over the DHSS limits.

Table 10.13
Charge registration officers thought would be
reasonable (homes charging too much)

	N	%
90	3	8.8
95	1	2.9
100	10	29.4
105	2	5.9
110	2	5.9
115	2	5.9
120	2	5.9
125	6	17.6
130	1	2.9
140	1	2.9
Totals	30	100.0

Missing cases= 4

Homes charging too little

The seven homes considered to be charging too little had minimum charges between £12 and £55 less than the registration officer considered reasonable (mean £30.57). The minimum charge ranges from £0 and £75 less than the DHSS limit of £120 per week (mean £26.29). The charge that the registration officers considered reasonable varied from £100 to £160 per week (mean £124.29).

It is possible to use these data to calculate the financial consequences of employing registration officers to assess the reasonableness of charges on the assumption that all other things remain the same. The consequences vary according to the parameters within which registration officers might work. Table 10.14 summarises the results. First the table gives the weekly cost of paying either the charge or £125, whichever is less, for one person in each of the 222 homes in the sample. This is £25,285 per week. If the homes charging too much had their charges lowered to what the registration officers considered reasonable or the DHSS limit, whichever was less, £3,700 would have been saved or 14.6 per cent of expenditure (on minimum charges). If in addition the charges of those homes charging too little were raised to what the registration officer considered reasonable or the DHSS limits, whichever was less, the net saving would be £2,895 per week or 11.4 per cent of total expenditure. Alternatively if national limits were abolished and the DHSS paid all charges at the level the registration officers considered reasonable, expenditure would increase - by only £376 per week - 1.5 per cent.

Table 10.14
Cost/savings of Registration Officers' recommendations

£ per week

1. Existing costs of B & L charges at charge
    or £125 if charge is greater   £25,285 (N=222)

2. Homes charging too much, minimum charge
    lowered to what registration officer
    considers reasonable or £125 whichever
    is less   -£3,700 (N=34)

3. Homes charging too little, minimum charge
    raised to what registration officer
    considers reasonable or £125 whichever
    is less   £805 (N=7)

4. Both 2 and 3   -£2,895 (N=41)

5. All homes charges paid at the minimum
    registration officers consider reasonable   £25,661 (N=222)

These calculations provide a general indication of the impact on SB expenditure of employing registration officers to fix charges. They indicate that between 10-15 per cent of total expenditure could be saved if registration officers worked within a framework of national limits. Relying on registration without a framework of maximum limits would have a very small impact on overall expenditure.

Obviously further work on these estimates is required. As they stand they must be viewed as the starting point for discussion rather than firm conclusions. In their present limited form the estimates of costs/savings from adopting 'reasonable charges' assume no supply response from the private sector. If reasonable charges were subject to limits the scope for private sector profits would be reduced. Given time, supply in the private sector might fall, or increase less quickly than otherwise. Although outcomes such as these might be predicted from a theory of elementary market behaviour it is unclear whether, in reality, home owners would respond in this way. If national limits failed to yield acceptable profits homes might well undertake intense marketing to attract a greater number of financially independent residents thus reducing their reliance on residents receiving public funds. In this account the supply of places for some residents would fall, or increase less quickly, but would be counterbalanced by moves to attract other groups of residents. A number of other responses are also available to home owners before any decision on their part to sell in order to cut losses.

If private homes chose to offer fewer places to SB claimants the immediate effect would be at least a slowing down, and possibly an absolute reduction, in SB expenditure. However, those judged in need of care will not go away. If their need cannot be met by the private sector, local authorities will be required to support them in the community or provide accommodation for them in their own Part III or Part IV homes. Although SB expenditure might fall other areas of public expenditure would increase.

We also indicated that, other things being equal, there would be a slight increase in SB expenditure if national limits were set aside and DHSS paid all charges considered reasonable. Again, some form of response from home owners is likely, possibly an increase in the proportion of places for SB residents. Such a response will, or course, have further implications for SB expenditure in this area.

Factors taken into account

Table 10.15 provides a summary of the reasons given by the registration officers for finding the charge unreasonable. There are two messages from this table - in some cases registration officers consider the facilities were inadequate for the charge. In other cases what is important is that, comparatively, the charge is higher than homes of an equivalent standard elsewhere. In short, their judgements were influenced by both absolute and relative considerations.

Table 10.15
Reasons given for finding the charge was unreasonable

		N	%
1.	Facilities are inadequate for the charge	15	30.6
2.	Home provides inadequate minimum standards	4	8.2
3.	Multi-occupancy of rooms/bed number too high	3	6.1
4.	Poor staff attitude/training/high turnover	3	6.1
5.	Charge based on physical amenities rather than on quality of care	2	4.1
6.	Charges are above the average	9	18.4
7.	Owner only takes active elderly - less mobile asked to leave	1	2.0
8.	Home is institutionalised	2	4.1
9.	Charges maximum available rather than for services/facilities provided	3	6.1

Table 10.16 provides a summary of the relative influence of different factors in making a judgement about the reasonableness of charges. In considering the home itself, the registration officer's judgement of the quality of care, the atmosphere within it and the presence of experienced staff were all more influential factors than the physical characteristics of the home, its location and the standard of catering.

There was little difference in the factors that were taken into account between those charges assessed as reasonable and those charging too much.

In comparison with those things associated with the homes, other factors that might have influenced the judgement were less important. Thus the state of the local market was a great influence in only 15 per cent of cases and no influence in 42 per cent. Charges in the public sector homes in the area were a great influence in 17 per cent of cases and no influence in 32 per cent of cases. In their briefing the registration officers were explicitly asked not to take account of the finances of the residential home owner and in 93 per cent of cases they did not. However in 15 cases the registration officers said the home's finances were some influence and in one case it was a great influence. There were some smaller homes providing a high quality of care where the registration officers admitted to being concerned about their viability and the need to keep a stable roof over residents even if the charges were too much.

There is evidence (not statistically significant) that these three factors which are not related to the character of the home were more important influences in the cases where the charge was considered unreasonable. In each case (see Table 10.16) a larger proportion of those who considered the charges for the homes were too high took some account of the state of the local market, charges for Part III and Part IV accommodation and the finances of the residential home owners.

In addition to the range of possible comparative factors discussed above, registration officers were also asked about the possible influence of current limits on their judgements. The consensus of opinion was that existing limits had no, or at most, minimal influence - with the observation from registration officers in two areas that ordinary board and lodgings rates were a more important influence. They tended to assess whether the care element provided by the homes was worth the difference between the charge and the normal board and lodging limit. Asked about the adequacy of £125, assessors in Lothian felt it was slightly below what was required for operating a 'good' home. The rest felt is was adequate, with the proviso from Devon that it was perhaps not quite enough to ensure adequate standards in smaller homes. Questioned about the influence of the earlier local limits, registration officers in three areas where these had been above the present £125 claimed that this had not influenced their decision about reasonableness of charges. The one area where the previous limit had been below the current one, felt this had influenced their decision.

Table 10.16
Influence of different factors in making judgements about reasonableness of charges

	No influence %	Some influence %	Great influence %
Local area	7.7	76.6	15.8
Upkeep of garden and exterior of property	12.6	80.2	7.2
Decorative order and standard of furnishings	5.9	73.4	20.7
Range and quality of facilities	4.1	48.6	47.3
Presence of experienced staff	6.3	38.3	55.4
Quality of care	4.5	27.9	67.6
Atmosphere within the home	6.3	36.0	57.7
Catering	2.7	78.4	18.9
State of the local market	41.9	43.2	14.9
Charges for Part III/IV homes	31.5	51.4	17.1
Finances for residential home owner	92.6	7.0	0.5

% saying it was some influence

	Charges reasonable	Charges too much	
State of local market	54.7	73.5	NS
Charges for Part III/IV homes	67.4	70.6	NS
Finances of residential home	5.7	14.7	NS

The judgements made by the registration officers in Lothian were rather different from those in other areas. They had access to the schedule of minimum charges that had been determined by their finance officers for sponsoring places in the independent sector. These as we have explained were based on a scrutiny of the accounts of each home that had been carried out annually but were now being uprated by an index. Although homes in Lothian had rather higher charges than elsewhere they were below their finance officers limits and this influenced the registration officers there in finding that only three of their homes were charging too much.

There is further evidence of the nature of the judgements being made in Table 10.17. The homes charging too much were much more likely to be rated overall as adequate or poor and to have lower rating scores. In those seven homes that were rated good or very good and yet were still considered to be charging too much, the judgement appeared to be a comparative one mainly with the facilities and charges in Part III/IV accommodation.

Table 10.17
Reasonableness of charges by overall assessment of home

| | Reasonable | | Too much | | Too little |
	N	%	N	%	N
Poor	2	1.1	9	26.5	—
Adequate	32	17.7	18	52.9	1
Good	74	41.4	6	17.6	2
Very good	62	34.3	1	2.9	3
Excellent	10	5.5	—	—	1
Totals	181	100.0	34	100.0	7
Rating Score Mean (SD)	26.1 (4.3)		20.1 (4.8)		28.0 (4.7)

x^2= 70.63   P<0.0001

The nature of the comparisons being made are shown in the next three tables. Table 10.18 shows that the facilities of those homes with reasonable charges are predominantly the same or better than other independent or local authority homes in the area and their charges tend to be the same or less than other homes. Table 10.19 shows that where their facilities are worse than other homes their charges tend to be less in compensation and where their charges are more than other homes their facilities tend to be better in comparison.

Table 10.18
Comparison of the assessed homes with others in the area

Comparison with other independent homes in the area

Facilities	Worse	Same	Better
Charges reasonable	25	82	71
Too much	24	5	4
Too little	–	2	5

Charges	Less	Same	More
Charges reasonable	53	98	25
Too much	6	17	10
Too little	1	2	4

Comparison with local authority homes in area

Facilities	Worse	Same	Better
Charges reasonable	32	54	90
Too much	25	5	4
Too little	0	2	5

Charges	Less	Same	More
Charges reasonable	90	45	43
Too much	7	8	19
Too little	3	2	2

Table 10.19
Comparison of the assessed homes with others
in the area: Charges judged reasonable

Comparison with other independent homes in the area

Facilities

Charges	Worse	Same	Better
Less	11	15	28
Same	13	57	28
More	–	8	16

Comparison with local authority homes in the area

Facilities

Charges	Worse	Same	Better
Less	14	24	50
Same	11	19	15
More	7	11	25

In contrast those homes charging too much tend to have worse
facilities than other homes and charge the same or more than
other homes. Where the homes charging too much (see Table
10.20) are charging the same or less than other homes their
facilities tend to be worse and where their facilities are
better than other homes they are charging more. There are only
four cases where the charges are the same or less than other
homes and the facilities the same.

Table 10.20
Comparison of the assessed homes with others in the area: Charges judged excessive

Comparison with other independent homes in the area

Charges	Facilities		
	Worse	Same	Better
Less	5	1	-
Same	14	3	-
More	5	1	4

Comparison with local authority homes in the area

Charges	Facilities		
	Worse	Same	Better
Less	5	2	0
Same	8	0	0
More	12	3	4

Finally, we asked registration officers whether they took into account different levels of dependency when making a decision about the reasonableness of charges. Some did, others did not. Devon, for example, thought that homes who took residents in particularly vulnerable conditions deserved more and encouraged them to seek registration for those categories which attracted a higher limit. Clwyd, on the other hand, did not feel that fees needed to be different for confused elderly people in a home with a mix of dependency. Sefton thought that a home should be a home for life and homes should cope with increasing dependency without increasing charges. Charges in Lothian were not judged in relation to the dependency of the residents though it was thought that charges for the elderly mentally ill were justified in being higher.

Method and timing of assessment

As we have already said the registration officers relied predominantly on their existing records, particularly those derived from the last registration inspection. However, over a quarter supplemented these with telephone calls to the home and in four per cent – nine cases – the home was actually visited. Registration officers confirmed that their own records contained a list of charges for each home, updated at each annual inspection.

The registration officers were also asked to make an estimate of the time taken to carry out the assessment and this is set out in Table 10.21. Where the assessment was based on existing records, in fact, the majority of cases, they estimated that on average it took 49 minutes. For the handful of cases where a visit was necessary, the assessment took over two hours to complete, with an hour at least taken up by travelling.

Table 10.21
Sources of information and time taken to make assessment

	% using method	Mean time spent minutes	(SD)	N	
Existing records from last inspection	99	43	(20)	219	
Phone calls	28	11	(7)	62	
Visit to the home	4	67	(24)	9	
Discussion with owner	6	23	(15)	11	
Overall mean		49	(24)	221	
Private		49	(21)	178	
Voluntary		52	(37)	43	
Charge reasonable		48	(25)	180	
Too much		55	(19)	34	NS
Too little		46	(19)	7	
Lothian 1		50	(47)	18	
2		26	(25)	17	
Devon 1		24	(3)	31	
2		40	(8)	15	
3		36	(14)	27	
Sefton 1		63	(4)	20	
2		70	(8)	22	
3		68	(14)	17	
4		71	(12)	27	
Clwyd 1		51	(9)	27	
Lothian		38	(40)	35	
Devon		32	(12)	73	
Sefton		68	(11)	86	$p < 0.001$
Clwyd		51	(9)	27	

137

There was little difference in the time taken to assess private and voluntary homes but those assessed as charging too much took rather longer than the others. There was considerable difference in the time taken by the different registration officers - thus Sefton 4 took an average of 71 minutes compared with only 24 minutes by Devon 1. In general the registration officers in Devon and one in Lothian carried out their assessments more quickly than those in the other areas. The variation in the amount of time required, and differences in registration officers' judgements, again has substantive implications similar to those raised in the assessment study. In short, the outcomes faced by home owners will depend on who happens to inspect them.

When we asked registration officers to say how they had completed our questionnaire, those in authorities outside of Sefton told us they worked on an individual basis. In Sefton, where the functions of registration and inspection are carried out by different officers, two registration officers worked together, and, likewise, two inspection officers. In retrospect they acknowledged that a better arrangement, and one reflecting their normal working practice, would have been for the pairs to contain a registration officer and an inspection officer each.

11 Discussion of charges study

Mechanisms for controlling charges

There are three possible mechanisms for controlling charges in independent homes.

The first involves procedures similar to those developed in Lothian for fixing maintenance rates for residents in private and voluntary homes. Proprietors of private homes and treasurers of voluntary homes are invited to submit their audited accounts and estimated costs for the following year on a standard form to the local authority. These are considered by finance officers, and after discussion with the homes, a maintenance charge is agreed. However, the process is lengthy, sometimes taking as long as three months from the submission of accounts. Whilst such an arrangement worked tolerably well when Lothian were supplementing people in the independent sector, it is likely to meet considerably more resistance from home owners in the much larger private sector outside of Scotland. Moreover, there is reason to question whether charges should be determined by cost or what the market can bear. Charges could be fixed on the basis of a home's costs including some reasonable return on the capital invested but a judgement would still have to be made about whether the resultant charge was reasonable to be paid from public expenditure given the local market and also whether the charge was reasonable given the standard of care provided.

The second involves the setting of limits. One form seeks to link the level of benefit to the type of care received by the claimant; national limits have also been applied, as have ones that reflect local variations. The Joint Working Party were in favour of the amount of benefit being set home by home but accepted that the amount would have to be for practical considerations, 'assessed locally within ceilings prescribed by DHSS nationally or regionally....'

The third option is to set aside costs and other charges relating to the capital invested in the home and consider the fees charged in relation to the facilities and quality of care provided, in comparison with other homes in the area and the state of the local market.

Can registration officers assess reasonableness of charges?

In the pilot study registration officers were able to make judgements about the general reasonableness of charges for homes in their area. How they viewed the task, and what implications they saw for their future role, is an issue considered later. Given that registration officers work closely with a limited number of homes, they soon acquire a comprehensive knowledge about them. They collect, at each annual inspection, a range of quantifiable information about the facilities and other physical features of a home. In addition, they will form strong impressions about other, less tangible, but equally important, aspects of the home such as the quality of care and quality of life. Other things being equal, it would seem but a small step to ask them to employ this knowledge and experience as a basis for making judgements, and advising local DHSS offices, about the level of charges it would be reasonable for supplementary benefit to meet in particular cases.

In real life registration officers may not be asked to make judgements about the general level of charges in a home as they have done in this study. They may have to make more precise ones that take into account the charge to an individual in a home. In order to do this they will need to bear in mind the charge in relation to the room and other facilities that may vary within a home. This would not be necessary for every home. In some the minimum and maximum charges are the same for the type of room, and in 30 per cent of homes the same even for different types of room. Such circumstances would certainly aid the registration officer's task by reducing the number of variables that have to be taken into account. However, in those homes where minimum and maximum charges are different for the same and different types of room, over half the homes in the study, the task would be more complex.

These points are based on the assumption that DHSS local offices will want a fresh decision about reasonableness of charges as each new claimant applies. A far more practical solution might be to agree the reasonableness of the charge home by home, and apply the answer to claimants en bloc. If so, the charge will need to be agreed with the proprietor as one aspect of the initial registration, subject, of course, to appeal and annual review.

Quality of care and the atmosphere within the home featured as the two criteria that had the greatest influence when registration officers formed a judgement about the reasonableness of charges. 'Home Life' attached considerable weight to these and other concepts such as privacy, autonomy, esteem and choice, but offered little advice on how they might be measured. However, these concepts are not intangibles and as such judgements can be formed even though the decision may be more difficult to make and less reliable than those concerning other physical features of the home. While judgements can be made about the underlying philosophy of care, and the tenets that give it substance, these 'soft' judgements might prove to be more open to interpretation and difficult to defend if contested. However, registration officers have to defend similar judgements at appeal when existing proprietors contest decisions to de-register and prospective owners challenge decisions which fail to provide them with initial registration.

The previous chapter considered the financial consequences of employing registration officers to assess the reasonableness of charges. The results indicated that at least 10 per cent of total expenditure might be saved if registration officers worked within a framework of national limits. Alternatively, if DHSS set aside national limits and allowed registration officers to fix the charge at the level they thought reasonable, there would be a marginal increase in expenditure. Both policy options have their strengths and weaknesses. The first would probably yield savings but would not entirely assuage the inflexibility and perceived inequity of the present system of national limits. Certain areas of the country would still feel hard done by. The second option would certainly introduce greater flexibility and respond to the criticisms levelled at national limits but has few financial attractions in terms of savings. Perhaps a third option is to allow registration officers to operate within a system of regional limits, the latter subject to regular review and updating. There are already special limits for London. However, there

are problems over variation within social security regions
where there exist areas of high charges and also areas of low
charges.

Possible implications for registration officer's future role

Among the registration officers who participated in this study
there were mixed views about whether it was appropriate for
them to take on the rôle of advising DHSS about the reasonableness of charges. It was not so much that they had doubts
about their qualifications for doing it though there was
anxiety about variation in officers' judgements and conflict
that might result. However more important was the possible
impact of the task on their existing duties. There were a
number of rather separate points. Registration officers see
their rôle as both inspectorial and advisory and rely on the
latter rôle to create a collaborative relationship with home
owners in order to work towards an improvement in standards.
Some felt that adding authority over-charges would ruin this
collaborative relationship. Instead of setting standards for
the home to work towards without responsibility for or control
of charges they might now be in a double bind with home owners
resisting improvements unless their limits were also lifted.
It was thought that in a local market comparisons would soon be
made between charges and facilities. Homes would withdraw
services if their charges were the same as another home not
providing it. It was even suggested that there would be great
temptation for registration officers to accept bribes from home
owners to get charges raised.

In contrast some of the registration officers felt that
taking on responsibility for recommending charges would enhance
their rôle by adding to the range of interventions they had.
It might lead in turn to a closer relationship between the
quality of the home and the level of charges that had been
found in this study. These officers felt that a working
relationship with the home owner could be too cosy. The kind
of judgements they would have to make and sustain were no
different to those made by for example the District Valuer.

It was also suggested that the high concentration of homes in
the four areas in our study meant that it was a rather
artificial basis for testing the capacity of registration
officers nationally to assess charges. In areas with very few
homes it would be much more difficult for registration officers
to make comparisons and build up experience in making
judgements.

There were also anxieties about the impact on their work load of fixing charges. This would be mitigated if charges were set at the annual registration visit - or set once and only increased in line with inflation unless the home owner could demonstrate that an increase was justified by improvements in services or facilities. Who would pay for the extra work involved? It was thought that the existing registration fee was not sufficient to cover the work involved in fixing charges and in Scotland no fee is payable by homes.

These are some of the issues and anxieties raised by the registration officers in the light of their experience during the project. In this study we have not explored the relative merits of different approaches and our results will need to be considered in the context of other studies that are currently taking a closer look at the costing of private residential care. It appears from the Lothian experience that involving financial officers in fixing charges has proved satisfactory. This study has shown that registration officers can also make judgements about whether charges are reasonable, without a detailed financial analysis based on the care being provided in exchange for the charge in comparison with other homes in the local market. It may be that in the end this assessment is the best and most cost-effective that DHSS could obtain.

Postscript

It is naturally too early to assess the impact of this research on policy. It was carried out to inform a Joint Central and Local Government Working Party. The Working Party chaired by Mrs Joan Firth published their report in July 1987. The report gave careful consideration to four options for harmonising the systems of financial support for residential care.

Option I - to transfer responsibility to the supplementary benefit system for all income support for residential care in both the public and independent sectors.

Option II - to give local authorities responsibility for financing all residential care costs which residents cannot meet themselves in both public and independent sectors.

Option III - in all sectors, to give responsibility to the DHSS for meeting the board and lodging element and to local authorities for meeting the care element in charges which residents cannot meet themselves.

Option IV - adapting the present system.

Each option was assessed on similar criteria. They concluded that if the present system continued there would be an unplanned drift involving increased numbers in residential care supported by supplementary benefits, withdrawal of local authorities in sponsoring places in the independent sector and a reduction in the number of places in local authority homes. There would also be continuing concern about whether people entering private homes needed that care and whether public resources were being used to best advantage. They therefore recommended that out of the alternatives, Option II was to be preferred. Local authorities would take over the assessment of need, the setting of standards and responsibility for all finance. This would help to control public expenditure, ensure value for money and encourage the development of domiciliary care and help target provision to the needs of the individuals.

On the issues of assessment of need and reasonableness of charges which were the central themes of the research the Committee were somewhat uncommitted and indeed divided. If Option I was to be introduced central government members did not feel that local authority assessment of need should be made a condition of entitlement to supplementary benefit. They felt that the evidence of the pilot studies "provide little support for the view that large numbers of elderly people were inappropriately placed in independent Residential Care Homes... Central government members did not believe that on the evidence so far, significant reductions in social security expenditure would result from introduction of a local authority assessment procedure which in itself would cost money... Those members believed that if Option I were to be pursued, further urgent study of the merits of assessment would be needed". para. 2.9.

On the other hand "local authority members were concerned to extend the advantages of a professional assessment procedure, which can inform and protect the individual, to all receiving public support for residential care and advocated early introduction of such a system". para. 2.10.

As the Committee came down in favour of Option II not Option I, this disagreement is not of great significance. Under Option II "Local authorities already assess the care needs of people for whom they provide residential care. Under Option II this assessment would be extended to anyone seeking financial support for residential care". para. 2.26.

On reasonableness of charges the Committee were impressed by our suggestion that to involve registration officers in fixing the reasonableness of charges would present them with conflicting roles. Local authority members felt that their staff could give advice on charges based on studies of the costs of homes but as far as Option I is concerned the

Committee saw "no alternative but to retain national limits set as sensitively as a national system can allow". para. 2.22.

If Option II (the preferred option) were to be pursued then charges would be left to local authorities to negotiate with individual home owners or places would be provided and priced through competitive tenders but there was no discussion in the report of what part registration officers might play in this process.

In the event Ministers have decided to delay making any decision on the report and have referred it to the health service policy adviser Sir Roy Griffiths who is conducting a review of community care and is due to report at the end of 1987.

The major problems with implementing the recommendation of the Firth Committee are likely to be political. It involves a substantial transfer of resources and control to local authorities. The Guardian (18 July 1987) commented "Mr Moore will have to sell this idea to Mrs Thatcher's cabinet which is certainly not in favour of boosting the role of local government" and "private home proprietors who were not present on the committee are unlikely to welcome the report".

PART III
ANNEXES

1 Pen pictures

Those requiring residential care at the time of admission but now able to cope outside with appropriate accommodation and support services

Case 1

Female, age 86, widowed

This woman was admitted to the present home in March 1986 after living alone in her own home. Her admission into residential care was initiated by hospital doctors and relatives, and she was assessed by a hospital doctor, social worker and professional staff before entry. On admission she was considered unable to manage in her own home after suffering from pneumonia. Since being in residential care her general condition has improved and it is considered that <u>warden-supervised sheltered accommodation</u> would be more suitable for her needs. This recommendation was made on the proviso that the resident would accept such a move and that accommodation of this type was available.

Case 2

Male, age 78, divorced

This man was admitted to the present home in March 1986 from his sister's home. His move was initiated by relatives and at the time of admission there were no differing perceptions about his need for residential care. On admission he was considered unable to manage in his own home and to need greater care and supervision than his sister could provide. Since being resident in the home his condition has improved and the Matron of the home feels he could physically manage in Warden-supervised sheltered accommodation although it is doubtful whether he would be prepared to move again now.

Case 3

Female, age 69, widowed

This woman was admitted to the present home in February 1985 after living in her own home. She suffered a stroke and was unable to manage independently so was admitted by a hospital social worker and was assessed by professional staff at the home as needing residential care. Her general condition has since improved although she has difficulties with speech and needs assistance to get in and out of the bath. The present home was assessed as being unsuitable for her needs and she was in the process of applying for sheltered housing.

Case 4

Female, age 85, widowed

This woman was admitted to the present home in January 1986 after living in her own home with her brother. Her move to residential care was initiated by her brother and a night nurse when her brother found he could no longer cope with caring for her. At the time of admission there were no differing perceptions about the woman's need for residential care but since then her condition has improved, with only physical help required getting in and out of the bath. It is felt that convalescent facilities or a short stay Rest Home placement (if available in the area) would have been preferable to immediate long-term care and breaking-up of the family home. Sheltered housing was judged to be a better alternative to the residential home in which she is currently placed.

Case 5

Male, age 81, married

This man was admitted to the present home in July 1986 after previously living in a private/voluntary residential home in another area. His spouse also lives in the home and at the time of admission it was only he who required residential care. Since being in the home his condition has improved and his wife intends to move them both to their own accommodation. Their names are on a council waiting list and she is considered to be able to care for herself and her husband.

Case 6

Female, age 90, widowed

This woman was admitted to the present home in March 1986 after living in her own home alone. Her move to residential care was initiated by relatives, and the local police assessed her to be in need of such care following a series of break-ins to her home. She agreed to move so as to alleviate the pressure on her family. Her general condition has improved slightly since being in the home, but it is considered that alternative accommodation would be more appropriate for her needs, ie. warden-supervised sheltered accommodation with appropriate support services such as home help or meals-on-wheels. It is felt that if a social work assessment had been done before admission then such alternatives would have been explored.

Case 7

Female, age 67, single

This woman was admitted to the present home in March 1985 following residency in a boarding house. A hospital consultant and GP advised her to leave the damp conditions of her flat and they assessed her to be in need of residential care. At the time of admission she was considered to be unable to manage in her own home because of the poor housing conditions, but during her time in the residential home her general condition has improved. She is now capable of living on her own and wishes to live independently, having kept her name on the sheltered housing list.

Case 8

Female, age 86, widowed

This woman was admitted to the present home in May 1986 after living with relatives. Her move into residential care was initiated by these relatives and she was assessed, by a general practitioner, local social worker and staff employed at the home, to be in need of such care. She was no longer able to live with her daughter as she (her daughter) was also caring for her terminally ill husband. At the time of admission she could not have managed on her own and her general condition since being in the home has stayed the same. The assessor has judged this woman to be capable of managing at home and has noted that her daughter has decided to take her back again.

Case 9

Male, age 72, single

This man was admitted to the home in January 1986 after living with relatives. He was referred to the home by a psychiatric hospital, the move initiated by a psychiatrist, hospital based social worker, relatives and the resident himself. At the time of admission there were no differing perceptions about the needs of this man, but now the resident feels he does not need the level of care provided by the home, although staff feel he could neglect himself if not supervised. His general condition over the period in the home has stayed the same, with supervision only required during bathing. Although the assessor believed the present home was not appropriate for the resident's needs, she felt that the matter was one for discussion and negotiation and that a supported landlady scheme would be a better alternative.

Case 10

Female, age 75, widowed

This woman was admitted to the home in November 1985 after living alone in sheltered housing. Her move into residential care was initiated by a hospital social worker and she was assessed by a hospital doctor, social worker and professional staff employed at the home as being in need of such care. The resident would have preferred to stay in her own home but was unable to cope and was medically at risk (diabetic) and the services needed to support her were either unavailable or overstretched. Although her general condition has improved slightly, the present residential home is considered suitable for her needs because she has become dependent on the home and could not manage on her own again. She believes that if she had known about available services earlier she would not have needed to move from her own home.

Case 11

Male, age 69, single

This man was admitted to the home in March 1986 after living with other people in his own home (squatters). His move into residential care was encouraged by a local area based social worker and professional staff employed at the home. At the time of admission he was considered unable to live at home because his house was uninhabitable, and although sheltered housing was seen as more appropriate, it was not available. Since being in the home his condition has improved, but he is still assessed as being unable to manage at home because his house has been sold.

Those not in need of residential care at the time of admission but now unable to cope outside even with appropriate accommodation and support services

Case 1

Female, age 81, single

This woman was admitted to the home in May 1986 after living in sheltered housing. Her move to residential care was initiated by herself and an assessment was made by a general practitioner and staff employed at the home. All concerned felt it was a good idea that she settle into residential care while she was fit and able to adjust and the home encouraged this move. Although she is still considered to be able to cope physically living in her own home, the assessor believed it unwise to move her now that she is so happily settled.

Case 2

Female, age 83, widowed

This woman Was admitted to the present home in November 1984 after living alone in her own home. Her move into residential care was initiated by herself with the support of friends/ neighbours, and an assessment of need was made by a general practitioner and professional staff employed at the home. It is possible that her move was fuelled by her anxiety about having further strokes after having already suffered one three years prior to admission. On admission it was judged that she could have managed at home for an estimated further two years. She appears to have no physical problems and it is only recently that she has become less mobile outside the home. She is now considered unable to manage in her own home – mostly for psychological reasons – because physically she would still just be able to cope. She is said to be very accustomed to life in the home and has no motivation to move.

Case 3

Female, age 90, widowed

This woman was admitted to the present home in January 1986 after residing in other residential homes since mid-1981. Relatives initiated her original move into residential care but she now feels she could have coped in her own home longer if she had been given time to get over her husband's death. Although her condition since being in the present home has improved she admits she has become dependent on the home and could not manage on her own again. She believes that if she had known about the available statutory services at the time, she could have got over her emotional shock and the fatigue of nursing her husband for five years, and could have coped on her own.

Case 4

Female, age 79, single

This woman was admitted to the home in December 1984 after living alone in sheltered housing. She made the decision to move into residential care herself because she felt she wanted to be looked after, so and no assessment was made of her needs.

Since being in the home her general condition has deteriorated, as she suffers from arthritis and she would no longer be able to cope, physically and psychologically, with living alone.

Case 5

Female, age 75, widowed

This woman was admitted to the present home in October 1984 after having lived in another residential home for two years. She required residential care because she had become homeless and felt she could not manage to set up home again. A general practitioner and professional staff employed at the home assessed her need for residential care. Her condition since admission has deteriorated (she is very deaf) and the assessor now considers that she would have difficulty in living alone again, although she would have managed in sheltered housing initially, if that had been available.

Case 6

Male, age 88, widowed

This man was admitted to the present home in August 1979 after living alone in his own home. His move into residential care was encouraged by his landlord who wanted to sell the house with vacant possession. The resident was unaware of alternative accommodation eg. sheltered accommodation, so initiated his own move into residential care and staff employed at the home assessed his needs. Although, initially he was considered able to cope alone and his condition has stayed the same since that time, it is now considered unlikely he would be able to cope on his own, as he has become accustomed to care and is happy where he is.

Case 7

Female, age 80, widowed

This woman was admitted to the present home in October 1984 after previously living in a boarding house/lodgings. She referred herself to residential care and was not assessed. After the death of her husband and brother she sought care and companionship, and now she is considered unable to cope on her own because her health has deteriorated during the time spent in the home. She feels that the present home is ideal for her needs.

Case 8

Female, age 72, widowed

This woman was admitted to the present home in March 1985 after living in the home of a friend whom she nursed. Following the deterioration in health of her friend, this woman chose to accompany her in to residential care rather than consider sheltered accommodation for which she was better suited. Her need for residential care does not appear to have been assessed at the time, although the assessor now believes she could not have coped alone without some general assistance. Although her condition has remained the same, the resident has become dependent on the care provided in the home and would not be able to live independently.

Case 9

Male, age 85, widowed

This man was admitted to the present home in December 1985 after living with relatives in his own home. He and his son aged 55 who has epilepsy, and has always been dependent on his parents, were admitted jointly. The father's need for residential care was not assessed and relatives initiated his move. At the time of admission, his niece considered that he could have managed at home with more suitable housing and support services, such as meals-on-wheels, if they had been available. Since his admission to the home his general condition has deteriorated, and now he would be unable to live independently.

Case 10

Male, age 55, single

This man was admitted to the present home in December 1985 after living at home with his father (see above). His admission was initiated by relatives and no assessment was made of his need for residential care. At the time of his admission he was considered to be able to cope at home, but only if rehoused with his father and given home help and meals-on-wheels. Although this resident's health has stayed the same, his father's condition has deteriorated rapidly. He has therefore been assessed as being unable to cope outside the residential home because he is dependent upon his father for general care and supervision, as he has been all his life.

Case 11

Female, age 74, widowed

This woman was admitted to the present home in May 1986 from another private/voluntary residential home where she had been unhappy. Her move into residential care was initiated by a general practitioner and her son and daughter, who also assessed her need for such accommodation. When first admitted to the home she was considered to be able to manage on her own although she suffered from depression following an illness. Since her time at the home her general condition has improved, but the assessor believes it would be too late to return her to living on her own, even with support services, because a disruption of her settled life now could make her depressed again.

Case 12

Male, age 79, married

This man was admitted to the home in January 1986 after living alone in his own home. His wife, from whom he is separated, also lives in the same residential home. His move to the home was initiated by himself and by relatives, but no assessment was made of his residential needs. On admission he was considered unable to manage on his own because his accommodation was poor and he was unable to look after himself, ie. budget for food and heating. The assessor felt it impossible to comment on the change in his condition since being in the home, but agreed that he would no longer be able to manage on his own because he has become used to being looked after. She also felt that an initial short-term arrangement and an assessment made of his options would have been better than an admission (at the time he was not on the social services files), as she thought social isolation had been his main problem.

Case 13

Female, age 82, single

This woman was admitted to the present home in January 1986 after living alone in her own home. She was given <u>notice to quit her rented flat</u> in 1985 and as she had no <u>family or friends locally to</u> support her, she felt a move into residential care would be best, although she could cope alone. She was assessed prior to admission by staff employed at the home and staff at the Housing Department. Prior to admission to the home, she had <u>requested sheltered accommodation</u> for which she felt better suited, but, as there were few options available, she turned to residential care. Since being in the home she has developed cancer and now requires care and emotional support. Although she may still be able to cope physically living alone, psychologically she needs support from the home.

Case 14

Female, age 79, widowed

This woman was admitted to the present home in October 1986 from another home where she had lived since September 1985. Before to that she lived alone in her own home. Her initial move into residential care was initiated/encouraged by the Baptist Church and an assessment of her needs provided by a general practitioner and professional staff employed by a voluntary organisation. At the time of admission to the first home, she was considered to be able to manage on her own at home for another 12 months, and she herself did not want to go into a home at that stage. She is blind and as her church felt she was not coping, arrangements were made for her admission to the first home. The assessor felt she <u>could have stayed at home with the assistance of home care</u>, but now, after being in residential care for over a year, feels she could probably not manage alone again, even though her general condition has not changed.

Case 15

Female, age 82, single

This woman was admitted to the present home in September 1985 after living in her own home with a spinster friend of 40 years. <u>A dispute with her friend</u> over money is given as the reason for her wish to go into care, although at the time of admission, she was considered to be able to live at home for another six months. A general practitioner and staff employed at the home assessed her need for residential care. During her time at the home, her condition has deteriorated and over the survey period she was in hospital because of repeated falls and dementia. She is definitely in need of care now, and her need for even more care is currently being assessed.

Case 16

Female, age 81, widowed

This woman was admitted to the present home in July 1986 after living alone in sheltered housing. She and her sons initiated her move into residential care and she was assessed by professional staff employed in the home. Her GP and the warden of the sheltered housing believed that she could have coped alone for some time - the warden considered that short-term care followed by a return to the sheltered housing would have been more appropriate. However her sons seemed to put pressure on her to move into residential care and since being in the home, her general condition has deteriorated (she suffers from depression), so that she is now considered unable to cope outside the home.

Those not in need of residential care at the time of admission and still not in need of it now

Case 1

Male, age 86, widower

This man was moved into the home from a privately rented flat as a result of his landlady's concern over his deteriorating eyesight and hearing in addition to an eight year history of 'heart trouble'. The admission assessment was made by his GP. He was not in receipt of ANY support services due to his lack of awareness both of their availability and his own eligibility and the general opinion appears to be that he could have been self-supporting - either in a home of his own or in sheltered accommodation if given the necessary back-up. However, although his general condition has remained stable since admission, he has no desire to attempt to cope on his own. The accommodation in the home is described as on a par "with a 5 star hotel" and in the subjects own words he "enjoys the best of both worlds" receiving a combination of care and freedom.

Case 2

Male, age 86, widower

This man was admitted after a self referral via a trade benevolent society. Having nursed his wife for twelve years until her death he left his own house in what is described as a "very exclusive area of Birmingham" feeling that after his prolonged efforts he wished to be cared for himself. The admission assessment was made by his GP. Prior to entry he was extremely independent, neither seeking nor requiring any assistance from relatives or available support services. It is apparent that he would be perfectly capable of managing in accommodation of his own and his condition has been maintained since entry.

NB. The home in question is the same as in the case above, and similar comments appear in both cases relating to the high standard. Both residents use this home as a "hotel" facility.

Case 3

Female, age 79, married

Since leaving their council house in Runcorn four years ago this resident and her husband, also resident, have led a "nomadic life", taking advantage of winter lettings at several coastal resorts, becoming homeless and then going into residential care when the accommodation was required for holiday makers. In this instance the husband needed medical attention and she entered care with him. Although she is capable of self-care she needs some assistance to cope with her husband. It is possible that the couple may move again, but it is obvious that at their age the wandering lifestyle is a poor substitute for a permanent home.

Case 4

Male, age 86, widower

Before entry to this home this man lived in _rented_
accommodation for fifteen years until his landlady developed
cancer and as a result sold the house. He was not in receipt
of, nor did he require the assistance of support services, and
he was fully independent up to the time when the house was
sold. His needs were assessed at the time of admission by
professional staff at the home. It is now suggested that
a sheltered housing scheme with mobile or ressistance from
relatives or available support services. It is apparent that
he _would be perfectly capable of managing_ in accommodation of
his own and his condition has been maintained since entry.

Case 5

Female, age 79, widow

Following the death of her husband this woman lives with her
son and his family for a period of ten years and as a result
neither required nor received formal support services. She
entered the home as a direct result of her son's divorce and
the sale of his house, and although both Housing Associations
and the local council were approached, because of the long
waiting lists there were no alternatives. Her needs were
assessed by the staff at the home. Despite needing some
physical assistance with bathing and use of the stairs she is
now seen as strong minded, preferring independence where
possible and being _capable of managing in sheltered_
accommodation where some assistance is available. A heart
condition and angina make it unlikely that she could live
independently in a home of her own.

Case 6

Female, age 83, married

Having cared for her husband in sheltered accommodation with
considerable support from formal services, this woman
moved with him into the home at a point where her family felt
she was unable to cope with his condition (unspecified) and she
agreed. The report indicates that she is "over anxious" about
her husband and, in consequence, separation would be highly
undesirable. Her own condition, barring a detached retina,
appears first class and her ability for self care is not in

question. As her husband's condition was deteriorating rapidly before entry it is apparent that he requires residential care and in the light of their relationship her obvious "best placement" is wherever he is.

Case 7

Female, age 69, separated

Despite some minor disablement from a hip replacement and a plate in one knee this woman is fully independent and perfectly capable of self care. She was forced to leave her flat in her husbands house at a point when his fixation with money led him to let every available space, including the cellar and use of her bathroom. She stayed for eight months in the home of one of her three daughters, but she felt "in the way" and left to enter the present home. She expects to be divorced shortly, and then this obviously strong willed woman intends to purchase her own flat in a sheltered scheme. In all probability she will not be in her present situation more than six months.

Case 8

Female, age 84, widow

This woman had housed a grand-daughter from an early age and after the girl's marriage had moved with the couple to their new home. Later, when they emigrated to South Africa, she went to live with her son and daughter in law in an unsatisfactory situation in which it appears she occupied the room of an adult grandson. This situation lasted four months at which point she was presented with a "fait accompli", her bags were packed for her and her entry into residential care apparently arranged and approved without her knowledge. Her needs were assessed by her GP and staff at the home. However, despite her obvious ability to cope (with support) in alternative accommodation, she has accepted her situation as being permanent, and any alternatives would be extremely difficult for her to accept.

Case 9

Male, 71, single

This man is an ex-merchant seaman (33 years) valet and butler. He is described as a former alcoholic of stubborn personality and has been diagnosed as suffering from terminal cancer of the pancreas. Although he has lived on his own for a short period in a council house, the majority of his life has been spent in situations where major services such as catering were provided for him. He moved into this home from a Veterans hotel when he realised that he would soon need more care than they could provide. In a few months it is likely that he will not be able to care for himself adequately and he does not have any contact with relatives who might provide support. His needs were assessed on admission by the GP and staff at the home.

Case 10

Male, age 81, widower

Following a stroke this man found the stairs of his "comfortable" third floor flat difficult to cope with, and he would have become lonely and isolated having always been an extremely active man. Although hospital staff did not feel he was in need of residential care and discharged him to his own home, he went to his daughter's home from where he entered this home. He was assessed on admission by the GP and stafff of the home. Although he might have managed physically in his own flat, emotionally life would have been difficult and his quality of life would have been of a lower standard than in this home which he obviously finds pleasant. He has had another minor stroke following his admission and feels frightened of any attempt to manage alone.

Case 11

Female, age 65, widow

This woman's main reasons for entry to the home are described as "homelessness and a desire to help others". She is obviously fit and active and independent in self care. Returning to Scotland from the USA where she lived with her husband until his death, she stayed temporarily with two incapacitated relatives on the Isle of Cumbrae but found she could not adapt to their inactive lifestyle nor cope with the somewhat primitive accommodation. Unable to find any suitable rented accommodation on the mainland she applied personally for a place in this home, and although settled at the moment, she may well find her trips to USA and to visit other relatives difficult to afford in the future, at which point it may seem less desirable. She was assessed on admission by the GP, social worker and staff at the home.

Case 12

Male, age 75, widower

Since his wife died in 1982 and he subsequently "fell out" with his youngest son, who left home, this man has been both depressed on his own but, more importantly, dismayed by his failure to obtain a smaller home despite being on the list for single persons sheltered accommodation for four years. However, he has not yet given up his own house, and at the time of the survey was obviously only in the home on a temporary basis as he was planning to return there two days after the interviews. He was assessed on admission by the GP and staff at the home, but it is possible that he only wanted a holiday and used the care facility to provide it. He was making sensible use of support services in his own home and perhaps should be considered as "passing through" rather than truly resident.

Case 13

Female, age 62, single

Having lived in an old council property that was poorly maintained and which suffered from drainage problems this woman made a concerted effort to get rehoused. Finally, vandalism and poor health increased her feelings of insecurity to a point where she applied for acceptance into residential care. She was assessed on admission by staff at the home. She is fully capable of self-care in a suitable environment and actively participates in such tasks as cleaning and helping the other residents within the home. Although a close relative was very much against her entry into care, she herself did not wish to burden her family and (perhaps realistically) sought the only credible alternative. She made virtually no use of support services while living at home.

Case 14

Male, age 88, widower

This independent man is fully capable of self-care, and gave considerable help to an invalid wife until her death eight years ago. He and his wife had lived in the same small council house for 18 years and had two daughters, now retired. Having observed other elderly person experiencing difficulties in self care and also in obtaining suitable accommodation when they could finally no longer cope, and realising the one daughter he would have liked to live with experiences ill health herself and would soon be unable to cope, he made a conscious decision to enter residential care before reaching crisis point. He was assessed by staff at the home and as he may well have become a client there anyway he merely pre-empted the event. He has a close friend already in the home and has ensured his future security to his own satisfaction. Because of his age the assessor found difficulty in placing him in the 'unsuitable' category.

Case 15

Male, age 75, widower

This man has a pacemaker and chest condition which causes him sporadic problems, and at these times he is very dependent. In the periods between these attacks he is extremely capable, and in consequence he would be an ideal candidate for supervised sheltered accommodation as living in the community without readily available 24-hour support is not a viable proposition. He has four sons, who are concerned, but unable to offer him accommodation and realising that remaining in his own five roomed flat alone was becoming an increasingly risky proposition he "put his name down" early so that help would be available when he needed it. He was offered a place more quickly than anticipated and entered the home for a trial period. He slipped into becoming a full-time resident and now regrets his decision to some extent, as he experiences boredom and restlessness and feelings of having "given a lot up". Suitable sheltered accommodation would have been a much more sensible and suitable alternative for him if it had been available.

Case 16

Female, age 72, single

This woman's blindness due to cataracts led to self-neglect including failure to maintain an adequate diet. She rejected offers of assistance from neighbours and the statutory and voluntary services available and was finally persuaded to enter a "rest home" by the landlady of her privately rented ground floor accommodation. Her need for residential care was assessed by the matron of the home and shortly after her admission all her furniture, etc. was sold. Now, having had her sight restored by successful removal of the cataracts, she is trapped in an environment she "dislikes intensely". Professional opinion is that she is capable of independent living for many years to come but is highly <u>unlikely to find suitable accommodation</u> in the area.

Case 17

Female, age 88, widowed

This woman was living on her own with some help from her son and daughter (in their 60s) before admission. The only service she requested was the district nurse, to help with bathing, but this was not available at the time. She planned her own admission because of her age, her need for some physical assistance and "everyones best interests". She wanted to make a decision while she "still had a choice" and did not wish to move into sheltered accommodation only to move again later on. While she is capable of independent living with some support services at the moment, it seems that she anticipated what would have been the inevitable outcome in the near future.

2 Assessment models

Two assessment models

Two models for assessment are outlined below. The first, from Canada, is an example of a working model that has been in operation since 1971; the second is again another working model based on recent research in Australia.

Model 1

Canada has one of the highest rates of residential care for old people in the world. However, many residents have been found to be inappropriately placed due to inadequate initial assessment (Chambers, et al., 1986). A Placement and Co-ordination Service (PCS) was established in Hamilton, Ontario in 1971 to remedy this situation. It is administered by a voluntary, non-profit making organization in the community and funded by the Ontario Ministry of Health. Its prime purpose is to facilitate, co-ordinate and centrally control the placement of elderly people. The PCS also seeks to promote better assessment and understanding of elderly people's needs and to make recommendations which take into account needs, wishes and available resources.

The three PCS counsellors, supported by two secretaries and an administrator, assist approximately 3000 clients each year. The counsellors do not carry out the assessments themselves. One form of assessment is completed by nurses and social workers using a standardized schedule that covers a wide range of demographic, social and functional items. The client's doctor completes a medical form covering diagnosis, prognosis, treatment, level of cognitive functioning and emotional status. Both forms are sent to the PCS who then act rather like a central clearing house, evaluating the material and making appropriate recommendations.

From their broad overview of the range of resources and services available the PCS is able to recommend not only different forms of institutional care but also rehabilitation, social and recreational programmes, home care housing, day care therapy centres and a number of other forms of community support. Rather than just keeping elderly people in the community the PCS's greatest achievement has been the development of reliable assessment measures which have significantly reduced the number of inappropriate placements.

The rationale, practice and results of the PCS are described in greater detail by Baynes and Caygill (1977), and by Baynes and Babiski (1978).

Model 2

Australia, like Canada, also places a large proportion of its elderly population in residential care. In fact 14 per cent of elderly people over 75 in Australia are in hospitals, nursing homes or old people's homes, twice the rate of the United Kingdom (Parker, 1985). Provision for the elderly tends to be uncoordinated, fragmented and undertaken by a diversity of private enterprises and numerous charitable and religious organisations. Against this background, and employing an action research approach, an Aged Referral and Assessment Unit operated as a pilot project for about 15 months in one part of the city of Sydney. The project hoped to demonstrate the advantages of a central referral agency for a variety of separate domiciliary support services. The idea of the central agency is akin to the PCS in Ontario, but avoids direct responsibility to a medical practitioner or geriatrician:

> While acknowledging that no assessment team could function effectively without access to the full range of geriatric diagnosis and medical care, the Unit operated on the

assumption that domination by health professionals may lead
to a one-dimensional view of multi-dimensional problems....

(Errey, et al., 1986, p.iv)

The philosophy stressed that assessment should be holistic in
nature, having regard to physical, psychological, social and
environmental factors. It was also important to view assessment
as an evolving rather than a 'one off' activity.

The Australian unit also differs from the Canadian PCS in so
far as its multi-disciplinary field staff undertook the
assessment of elderly people and worked with local groups to
deliver appropriate services. The Canadian counsellors performed
much more the role of an independent broker. Both schemes,
however, maintained extensive record systems including usage of
services and needs not met.

Comment

Both schemes have their attractions. The Canadian PCS, for
example, takes responsibility for making recommendations based on
the assessments forwarded to it by social workers and health
professionals, thus freeing them of this burden. Given the
number of staff involved, and the number of clients assisted, the
PCS would appear to be an efficient and cost-effective service.
The anxieties of social workers in this country about advising
DHSS local offices on a person's need for care might well be
allayed if an agency similar to the PCS were to evaluate their
assessment and make the necessary recommendation. It is less
certain whether British social workers would support the heavy
emphasis on health and medical factors in the PCS assessment. No
doubt in adapting the approach different emphases could be
introduced. One great advantage of adapting the PCS approach to
the British context is that it could embrace all forms of public,
private and voluntary care in residential as well as nursing
homes. It would certainly simplify matters if residential and
nursing home assessment procedures were similar, and processed by
the same central agency.

The concept of a central referral and assessment agency is
again at the heart of the Australian project, but with its multi-
disciplinary staff undertaking and evaluating their own
assessments. In the British context there may be good reasons
for keeping the two separate unless, of course, a degree of
'neutrality' could be ensured by not tying assessment teams to a
particular local government department or boundary. Although no
costings were available for the Australian scheme, given the

number of contact workers involved, and members of the assessment
team, it is likely to be much more expensive to operate than the
Canadian PCS. To some extent the extra costs will be counterbalanced by the savings that accrue from keeping elderly people
in the community rather than placing them in more expensive
hospital and other forms of residential care.

Bibliography

Audit Commission (1985), Managing Social Services for the Elderly More Effectively. London: HMSO.

Audit Commission (1986), Making a Reality of Community Care. London: HMSO.

Bayne, J. and Babiski, D. (1978), 'Identification by the Assessment and Placement Service of the numbers and care needs of ambulant confused persons', Canadian Journal of Public Health 69, 244-247.

Bayne, J. and Caygill, J. (1977), 'Identifying needs and services for the elderly', Journal of the American Geriatrics Society, 25(6), 264-268.

Bingley, W. (1986), 'Legal Eye', Care Concern, July/Aug., 14.

Booth, T., Barritt, S., Berry, S., Martin, D, Melotte, C. and Stone, S. (1982), 'Levels of dependency in local authority homes for the elderly', Journal of Epidemiology and Community Health, 36(1), 53-57.

Booth, T. and Berry, S. (1984), 'An overdose of care', Community Care, July 25, 22-24.

Brocklehurst, J., Carty, M., Leeming, J. and Robinson, J. (1978), 'Medical screening of old people accepted for residential care', Lancet, 2, 141-143.

Brooke-Ross, R. (1985), 'Regulation of residential homes for the elderly in England and Wales', Journal of Social Welfare Law, March, 85-95.

Butler, A., Oldman, C. and Greve, J. (1983), Sheltered Housing for the Elderly: policy, practice and the consumer, National Institute Social Services Library No. 44. London: George Allen and Unwin.

Carson, D. (1985), 'Registering homes: another fine mess?', Journal of Social Welfare Law, March, 67-84.

Centre for Policy on Ageing (1984), Home Life: a code of practice for residential care, Report of a working party, under the Chairmanship of Kina, Lady Avebury.

Challis, L. (1986), 'Robbing Peter to Pay Paul - handsomely', Social Services Insight, Aug. 16, 12-14.

Chambers, L., Haight, M. and Caygill, J. (1986), 'Evaluation of Placement and Coordination of Geriatric Services using a health program evaluation grid', Clinics in Geriatric Medicine 2(1), 137-150.

Charlesworth, A. and Wilkin, D. (1982), Dependency among Old People in Geriatric Wards, Psychogeriatric Wards and Residential Homes 1977-81, Research Report No. 6, University Hospital of South Manchester.

Cobb, J. (1978), 'Medical screening of old people', Lancet, 2, 676.

Coles, O. (1985), 'The dependency of old people in residential care: interpreting the trend', Social Services Research, 14(5), 37-66.

Davies, B. and Challis, D. (1986), Matching Resources to Needs in Community Care, Aldershot: Gower.

DHSS (1984), Population, Pension Costs and Pensioners' Income. London: HMSO.

DHSS (1985), Supplementary Benefit and Residential Care, Report of a Joint Central and Local Government Working Party, (Chairman: Mr Scott-Whyte).

DHSS (1987), Public Support for Residential Care, Report of a Joint Central and Local Government Working Party, (Chairman: Mrs Firth).

Errey, R., Baker, C. and Fox, S. (1986), Community Care of the Aged: A Working Model of a Needs-Based Assessment Unit, SWRC Reports and Proceedings No. 59, Social Welfare Research Centre, University of New South Wales.

Fryer, R.G. (1985), Implementation of the Registration Homes Act 1984 in Leicestershire, DHSS, Social Services Inspectorate.

Fryer, R.G. and Mountney, G.H. (1985), Inspection of a sample of residential accommodation for the elderly provided by the local authority and private sectors in Lincolnshire carried out during 1984/85. DHSS, Social Services Inspectorate.

Judge, K. and Sinclair, I. (eds.) (1986), Residential Care for Elderly People, Research contributions to the development of policy and practice. A collection of papers presented to a DHSS seminar in October 1983. London: HMSO.

Lowther, C. and McLeod, H. (1974), 'Admission to a welfare home', Health Bulletin, 32, 14-18.

Murray, N. (1986), 'A hung hybrid', Social Services Insight, Nov. 21, 12-14.

Neill, J. (1982), 'Some variations in policy and procedure relating to Part 3 applications in the GLC area', British Journal of Social Work, 12(2), 229-245.

Ovenstone, I.M. and Bean, P.T. (1981), 'A Medical Social Assessment of Admissions to Old Peoples Homes in Nottingham', British Journal of Psychiatry, 139, 226-229.

Parker, R.A. (1985), The growth of private nursing homes in Australia: The lesson for Britain. Department of Social Administration, University of Bristol.

Shipley, C. (1985), Report on information day - South-west region registered homes standing group at Crossmead Centre, Exeter 16.5.85. DHSS, Social Services Inspectorate.

Stapleton, B. (1977), 'A survey of the waiting list for places in Newham hostels for the elderly', Clearing House for Local Authority Social Services Research, 5, 29-60.

Tibbenham, A. (1985), Private and Local Authority Care of the Elderly in Devon. Devon County Council, Social Services Department Research Section.

Tinker, A. (1984), Staying at Home: Helping Elderly People, London: HMSO.

Watson, R. (1986), 'Phenomenal growth in private care for the elderly poses a challenge', Municipal Review, No. 664, 181-182.

Weaver, T., Willcocks, D. and Kellaher, L. (1985), The Business of Care: a study of private residential homes for old people. Centre for Environmental and Social Studies in Ageing, Polytechnic of North London.

Whitehouse, A. (1983), 'Beveridge could not have been more wrong', Community Care, April 28, 14-16.

Willcocks, D., Peace, S. and Kellaher, L. (1982), The Residential Life of Old People: A study in 100 local authority homes, Polytechnic of North London, Department of Applied Social Studies – Survey Research Unit Reports No. 12 and No. 13.

Index

housing benefit 81
income other than SB 75

Joint Central and Local
   Government Working Party
   vii, 5-8, 93-95, 144-146

Joint Unit for Social Services
   Research 7,

Kent Community Care Scheme 81,
   84

legislation 96-97
   criticisms of 97
   Nursing Homes Act 1975 96
   Registered Homes Act 1984 5,
   9, 95, 103
   Registered Homes Tribunals
   1984 96
   Residential Care Homes
   Regulations 1984 96
   Social Work (Scotland) Act
   1968 9, 95, 103

Local Authority Associations
   5, 6

Lothian Regional Council
   revenue account 10n

Lowther, C. 6

McLeod, H. 6

mobility allowance 74

Modified Crighton Royal (MCR)
   Scale 43-49

Mountney, G. 4

Murray, N. 12, 99

Neill, J. 43

Ovenstone, I. 6

Parker, R. 168

participating authorities-
   see 'pilot areas'

pen pictures of residents 22-
   23, 149-166

personal allowance 78, 81

Personal Social Services
   Statistics 10n

pilot areas,
   Clwyd 10, 13
   Devon 10, 11-12
   Lothian 9-11
   Sefton 10, 12

Population Estimates Scotland
   10n

Quarterly Statistical Enquiry
   3

rating of the home,
   and actual charges 116-118
   factors taken into account
   113
   and overall assessment 114
   raw and weighted scores 114
   variation 115-116

reasonableness of charges,
   and actual charges 124
   and dependency levels 136
   homes with reasonable
   charges 125
   homes charging too much
   125-127
   homes charging too little
   127
   and overall assessment 133
   in pilot areas 122-123

reasonableness of charges
study,
   characteristics of homes
   105
   existing records of homes

103, 136–137
occupancy rates in homes
106–107
purpose 93–94
questionnaire 103–104
sample of homes 101–102
time required 136–138

registration officers 95–96
ability to assess charges
140
background and experience
100
financial consequences of
employing to assess charges
127–128, 141–142
general duties 98–100
influence on judgements 129–
133
response to assessing
charges 142
role in the research 100

residential care,
appropriateness and need for
5, 8, 37–40
categories of need 7, 15, 37
cost of alternatives 81–82
disputes over need for 58
options for harmonizing
financial support 144–146
process of admission 54–57
reasons for admission 49–51
recommendation for 66
staying out of 38
suitability 79
variations in need for 40–42

residential care homes
number nationally 5
number in pilot areas 9–13
number of places nationally
3
local authority, private and
voluntary 3–6

resources,
effective use of 5
targetting 7, 82

sample,
areas – see 'pilot areas'
characteristics of
claimants 20–24, 68–79
selection of claimants 14–
18

Scottish Office Library 10n

Scott Whyte Committee – see
Joint Central and Local
Government Working Party

services,
received 52–53
required 54–55

sheltered housing 24, 39, 52,
55

Shipley, C. 99

Social Services Inspectorate
4

social worker assessors,
background 33–34
reflections 34–36

sponsorship 5, 94

Stapleton, B. 43

'substitution effect' 89

supplementary benefit for
residential care,
adequacy of limits 131
average payment 4
and care assessment 84
claimants current SB status
74
claimants previous SB
history 72–74
escalation in payments 7
influence of limits on
charges 95
influence of limits on
registration officers'